Focus on Antipsychotics

Ben Green

For Clare

Focus on Antipsychotics

Ben Green

Consultant Psychiatrist and Honorary Senior Lecturer

Cheadle Royal Hospital and The University of Liverpool

REVISED EDITION

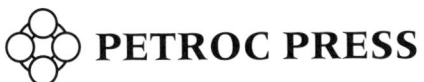 PETROC PRESS

Petroc Press, an imprint of LibraPharm Limited

Distributors

Plymbridge Distributors Limited, Plymbridge House, Estover Road, Plymouth PL6 7PZ, UK

Copyright

© LibraPharm Limited 2002

All rights reserved. No part of this publication may be reproduced, stored in a retrieval system, or transmitted in any form or by any means, electronic, mechanical, photocopying, recording or otherwise, without prior permission from the publishers.

While every attempt has been made to ensure that the information provided in this book is correct at the time of printing, the publisher, its distributors, sponsors and agents, make no representation, express or otherwise, with regard to the accuracy of the information contained herein and cannot accept any legal responsibility or liability for any errors or omissions that may have been made or for any loss or damage resulting from the use of the information.

First edition 2002
Revised edition 2004

Published in the United Kingdom by

 LibraPharm Limited

Gemini House
162 Craven Road
NEWBURY
Berkshire
RG14 5NR
UK

A catalogue record for this book is available from the British Library

ISBN 1 900603 58 6

Typeset by ReadyText Publishing Services, Bath
Printed and bound in the United Kingdom by MPG Books Ltd, Bodmin, Cornwall PL31 1EB

Contents

About the Authors		vi
Foreword		vii
Chapter 1	Introduction	1
Chapter 2	Antipsychotic Development: the Historical Record	4
Chapter 3	ECT: an Effective, but Ignored, Treatment of Psychosis	10
Chapter 4	Prediction of Response to Lithium in Affective Disorders	18
Chapter 5	Focus on Chlorpromazine	24
Chapter 6	Focus on Haloperidol	29
Chapter 7	Focus on Clozapine	37
Chapter 8	Focus on Risperidone	45
Chapter 9	Focus on Olanzapine	53
Chapter 10	Focus on Quetiapine	60
Chapter 11	Focus on Amisulpride	66
Chapter 12	Focus on Ziprasidone	71
Chapter 13	Focus on Depot Antipsychotics	76
Chapter 14	Antipsychotics in the Elderly	79

About the Authors

Dr Ben Green MRC Psych, MB, ChB, ILTM
Honorary Senior Lecturer in Psychiatry, University of Liverpool, UK and Consultant Psychiatrist, Halton Hospital, Cheshire, UK.

Address for correspondence:

University Department of Psychiatry
Royal Liverpool University Hospital
The University of Liverpool
Liverpool
L69 3GA
UK

E-mail: bengreen@liverpool.ac.uk

Dr Samuel Vovnik MRC Psych, MB, ChB
Consultant Psychiatrist
University Hospital Aintree
Liverpool
UK

Dr David Healy
North Wales Department of
  Psychological Medicine
University of Wales College of Medicine
Bangor
LL57 2PW
Wales

E-mail: healy_hergest@compuserve.com

Professor Max Fink MD
Professor of Psychiatry and Neurology Emeritus, School of Medicine, SUNY at Stony Brook; and Professor of Psychiatry, Albert Einstein College of Medicine.

P.O. Box 457
St. James
New York 11780
USA

Tel: 631.862.6651
Fax: 631.862.8604
E-mail: mafink@attglobal.net

Dr M T Abou-Saleh MB, ChB, MPhil, PhD, FRC Psych
Reader in Addictive Behaviour
Department of Addictive Behaviour and
  Psychological Medicine
St George's Hospital Medical School
Cranmer Terrace
London
SW17 0RE
UK

Prof. Dr. Borwin Bandelow
Dept. of Psychiatry
The University of Goettingen
Robert-Koch-Str. 40
D-37075 Goettingen
Germany

Tel: +49-551-396607
Fax: +49-551-392004
E-mail: bbandel@gwdg.de

Dr Miriam Naheed MRC Psych
Specialist Registrar
Hollins Park Hospital
Winwick
Cheshire
UK

Dr Emad Salib MB, DPM, MSc, MRCPI, FRC Psych
Honorary Senior Lecturer, Liverpool University and Consultant Psychiatrist, Hollins Park Hospital, Warrington.

Foreword

Professor Richard Morriss

Antipsychotic drugs remain a lynch pin of the armamentarium of the psychiatrist. These drugs revolutionised the outcome for patients with serious mental illness, particularly schizophrenia, enabling many thousands of patients to live outside institutions when previously they would have remained in institutional care for most of their lives. Antipsychotic drugs clearly have been enormously beneficial to patients and cost-effective to society, when prior to 1960 one quarter of all beds in the British National Health Service were occupied by patients with schizophrenia. The identification of chlorpromazine and the widespread use of antipsychotic drugs in the late 1950s onwards, together with the political decisions to concentrate care in the community in many of the developed countries, were associated with large reductions in the numbers of medium- and long-stay hospital beds occupied by patients with schizophrenia. Antipsychotic drugs have also been frequently used to treat mania, agitation and psychotic symptoms in patients with depression and dementia.

Nevertheless, antipsychotic drugs have caused patients to have side-effects and in some instances these have had a serious adverse effect on the patients' quality of life. Over the last decade there have been many notable developments in the management of patients with schizophrenia. These include the development of new antipsychotic drugs, the realisation that conventional neuroleptics were often just as effective with fewer side-effects at lower dosages than at higher dosages, the dangers of sudden death from some antipsychotic drugs, the introduction of effective psychological treatments, such as cognitive behaviour therapy and family therapy, and more effective models of service delivery such as assertive community treatment. The benefits of such progress in management has enabled the psychiatrist to refine their treatment options and tailor them more effectively to the individual circumstances and mental state of each patient. The increasing demands for such an approach from patients and carers, and scepticism about doctors, require the psychiatrist to know considerably more about the antipsychotic drugs they use. The psychiatrist in the present day also has to have a clear picture of the precise role of antipsychotic drugs as part of a general package of care.

Hence this book is timely because it contains a wealth of factual information on both typical and atypical antipsychotics plus chapters on ECT and lithium that are frequently used alongside antipsychotic drugs. Included is the background to the development of antipsychotics and the clinical application of antipsychotics in the elderly. Psychiatrists will be able to consult this textbook for the detail they require and use this information to negotiate with their patients, carers and fellow health professionals a package of treatment, which is usually both effective and acceptable for all concerned.

Richard Morriss
Professor of Psychiatry
University of Liverpool
3rd August 2001

Chapter 1

Introduction

Dr Ben Green

This revised edition of Focus on Antipsychotics gathers together a number of review papers on modern antipsychotic agents.

The aim is to provide a concise and up-to-date source of evidence-based opinion regarding the drugs.

The customs and practice of prescribing vary very much from country to country, but I believe that this short volume covers the most popular antipsychotic drugs.

A small-scale survey of international psychiatrists indicates the 2001 preferences of psychiatrists for second-generation drugs – see Figure 1.1.

Risperidone is clearly identified as the leading prescriber preference, reflecting perhaps its wider availability and longer history. Chapters in this book cover all the drugs in Figure 1.1.

The case for the use of antipsychotics is a strong one. The lack of efficacy of and inhumanity of historical treatments has been well described. The societies and mad-doctors of previous centuries have relied on such methods of containment and therapy. For many years chains and frank methods of restraint were employed to hold people in houses of correction, prisons and workhouses (Figure 1.3).

Vast workhouses sprang up across Europe to house the poor, the old and the psychotic. Liverpool's workhouse was a small town within a city, warehousing some 5,000 individuals.

In the UK the county asylums were set up with philanthropic intentions of providing good clean air and a therapeutic environment providing occupations on the often-associated farms. The sometime quoted idea was to remove patients from the 'miasmas' of the city, which were thought to be important in the aetiology of psychotic illness. Asylums in one form or another had been available to smaller numbers

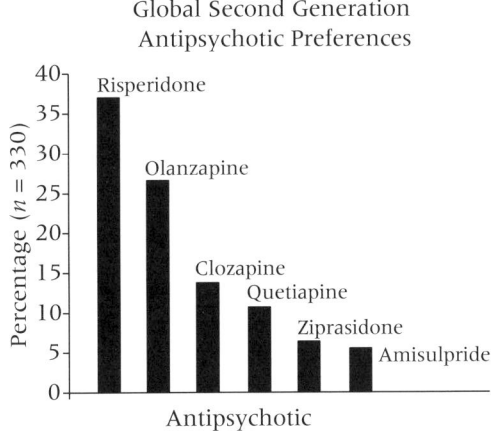

Figure 1.1: Summary of opinions of 330 psychiatrists answering an on-line professional poll in December 2001 regarding second generation antipsychotic preferences. Source: Psychiatry On-Line:
http://www.priory.com/psych.htm

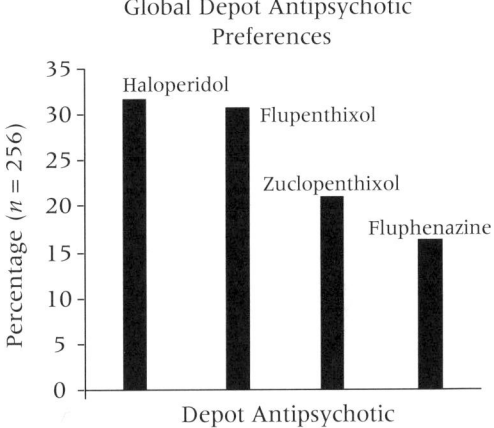

Figure 1.2: Summary of opinions of 300 psychiatrists answering an on-line professional poll in December 2001 regarding depot antipsychotic prescribing. Source Psychiatry On-Line:
http://www.priory.com/psych.htm

in hospitals such as the Bethlam Hospital in London since the thirteenth century (Figure 1.4). Hogarth depicted the hospital in his *Rake's Progress* and an uncomfortable place it looks with a cluttered mix of patients with grandiose or religious delusions wrestled with by mad-doctors and nurses and viewed as entertainment by paying visitors as if they were touring zoological gardens.

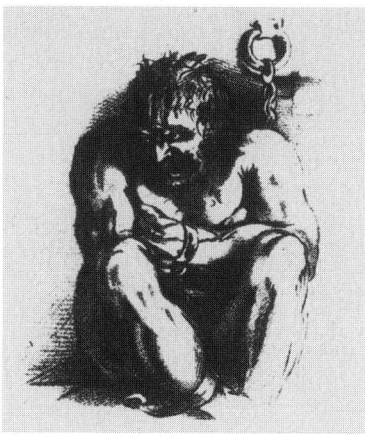

Figure 1.3: *The use of chains for security and containment. From* Madness, or a man bound with chains *by Sir Charles Bell (1774–1842). London: Longman, Hurst, Rees, and Orme, 1806. Reproduced with permision.*

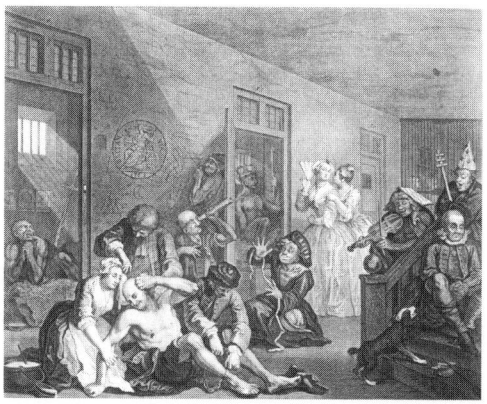

Figure 1.4: *Depiction of life in a ward at Bedlam in* The Rake's Progress *by William Hogarth (1697–1764). Reproduced with permission.*

Prior to the introduction of antipsychotics in the 1950s physicians flailed about trying to find suitable treatments that would reduce the intolerable human suffering that schizophrenia and other psychotic illnesses produced. Kraepelin's audit of clinical practices in the older hospitals indicated stays of decades for the majority of patients. This gloomy prognosis was typical for the psychotic disorders, no matter what treatment modality was employed whether it be talking therapies, hypnotism, Mesmerism, whirling chairs (Figure 1.5), asylums, wet blanket therapy or sundry other therapies borne more out of desperation than Scientific Method.

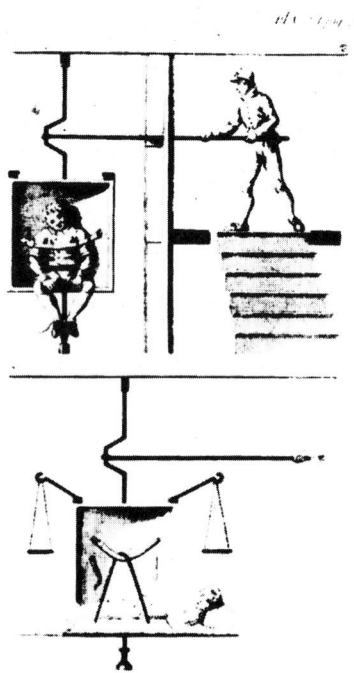

Figure 1.5: *The Whirling Chair – used in various forms in Europe and the USA to treat psychosis, with little effect. Illustrated in: Traité sur l'alienation mentale et sur les hospices des aliénes; Joseph Guislain, Amsterdam, Van der Hey, 1826. Reproduced with permission.*

The accumulation of patients with time seems clear in the public asylum records of the time (Table 1.1).

Table 1.1: *Total number of patients in public asylums in England and Wales.*

Year	Number
1850	7,140
1870	27,109
1890	52,937
1910	97,580
1930	119,659
1954	148,100
1960	136,200
1970	103,300
1980	92,000

The asylums, once established in a more widespread fashion in the UK in the late nineteenth century, promptly began to expand. The workhouses were slowly being closed, and insanity was seen as a 'medical issue'. Expansions of asylums varied between 1 and 10% per annum, leading to large asylums sized at 1–2,000 beds, such as Winwick and Rainhill Hospitals. At the inception of the UK National Health Service in 1948 half the UK hospital beds were for mental illness.

Reducing trends in the large number of psychiatric beds for psychosis only became possible following scientific advances, such as the identification and treatment of syphilis, the development of ECT, psychosurgery and insulin coma therapy. With the advent of antipsychotic drugs these other physical methods of treatment were practically all replaced, by virtue of the antipsychotics' superior efficacy and greater tolerability. The reduction in bed occupancy post-1950s – despite a burgeoning general population – seems clear enough in Table 1.1, and is attributable purely to the success of the first generation of antipsychotics.

Antipsychotic drugs have therefore made a considerable and lasting impact on the burden of mental illness for the individual and society. It is sobering to realize that despite the much-publicised areas of cognitive behavioural therapy, social policy and Care Programs, without antipsychotic drugs these methods of treatment would be no more effective than the whirling chairs and asylums of old.

Your feedback for future editions would be very welcome and can be addressed to me either at the postal or e-mail addresses listed in the front of this book.

Chapter 2
Antipsychotic Development: the Historical Record

Dr David Healy

The first steps

Traditional accounts of the discovery of chlorpromazine emphasize the serendipitous nature of what happened. In the context of the times, nothing could have been further from the truth. After the Second World War, Rhône-Poulenc and other companies were very deliberately in the business of producing anti-histamines. Rhône-Poulenc, in particular, stumbled on the fact that the phenothiazine molecule provides the basis for a number of anti-histamines. They set about systematically producing a series of phenothiazine anti-histamines. It became clear that these had central effects, leading the company to explore these actions of their new group of anti-histamines and to 'optimise' these.

But to what purpose were they optimising? The general notion was that these agents would be useful anti-stress agents. Stress in this context meant the physical stress of surgery or allergies. This led to an interest in producing a drug that would block as many 'ganglions' as possible. A ganglioplegic agent. Rhône-Poulenc wanted a drug that would target as many brain systems as possible in the belief that shutting down as many systems as possible was the best way to handle stress. It was these factors that led to the production of chlorpromazine. It was in this sense 'dirtier' than the other antihistamines. Dirty enough to be somehow 'antipsychotic', as it turned out[5].

Chlorpromazine was surprising in that it was in some sense a non-sedative sedative. Patients might appear asleep but could come out of this 'ataractic' state and interact in a manner quite unlike patients sedated with barbiturates or other sedatives. Even though patients were not sedated in the manner they had been sedated with the barbiturates, the consensus of opinion was that this drug was a sedative of some sort. A subsequent generation of drugs, therefore, aimed at being sedating. These included thioridazine, levomepromazine and clozapine, all of which had been produced by 1958[11,25,28].

The next breakthrough was the discovery in 1955 of the 'antipsychotic' properties of prochlorperazine[3]. This drug was not sedative. The example of prochlorperazine led to the notion that the new drugs worked by being neuroleptic rather than sedative. Common to both the sedative and the incisive ganglioplegics was a brain effect that mimicked the effects of encephalitis lethargica. The drugs produced motor problems, dyskinesias and dystonias as well as akathisia and by doing so, it seemed, benefited patients. The idea of a neuroleptic was born and this drove a desire to see less sedative agents, whose production of extrapyramidal effects was interpreted in a favourable rather than a problematic light.

The utility of the neuroleptic concept was dramatically demonstrated by the synthesis of haloperidol by Janssen. This drug was the first to breakaway from the phenothiazine nucleus. Chlorpromazine as it turned out could antagonise the effects of amphetamine on animals. Attempting to synthesise a new painkiller, Janssen and colleagues noticed that they had produced a series of compounds, which also antagonised amphetamine were not phenothiazines. They attempted to optimise the amphetamine antagonising properties of their new series and in the process produced haloperidol. The new agent was not sedative. It was effective at very low doses (1–5 mg)[12].

The next step was to attempt to produce a molecule that would antagonise both the behavioural effects in animals of amphetamines as well tryptamines, including LSD. This led in the early 1960s to the synthesis of dipiperone, also known as pipamperone. Dipiperone, as it turns out, is an effective D_2 receptor antagonist as well as a $5HT_2$ receptor antagonist[12]. But this

4

was not known at the time. In the changing climate of the 1960s, the somewhat sedative effects it had over and above haloperidol appeared to be a step backwards[26]. It failed in the market place.

Following the success of haloperidol, which became the best selling neuroleptic in the world, an antagonism of the varied effects of amphetamines and apomorphine in animal models became the method that directed the synthesis of new agents. Significantly, clozapine had been produced before this. Had the amphetamine model become dominant by the time clozapine was produced, it is probable that this molecule would have been shelved[20]. The amphetamine model mandated the development of drugs that produced catalepsy as well as drugs that blocked the effects of amphetamine in the production of a range of stereotypies. Clozapine had mixed effects on this range of tests.

From the mid-1960s, with the work of Carlsson and colleagues[1], and later Van Rossum[32], there was a move toward looking at the effects of these drugs on neurotransmitter systems. Carlsson's work emphasized the effects of the drugs on catecholamine systems in general, whereas van Rossum fingered the dopamine system in particular. It was not, however, until the early 1970s that attention began to focus clearly on the dopamine system. From 1971 to 1976, considerable international efforts went into establishing aspects of the pharmacology of the dopamine system[4,23]. Dopamine receptors were among the first to be radio-labelled, with the new techniques that were emerging in 1972/1973[22]. These approaches led to the discovery that there was more than one dopamine receptor. There were both D_1 and D_2 receptors. The antipsychotic agents preferentially bound to D_2 receptors. The doses of each of the then available agents that were needed to produce specific binding at this receptor site were also the doses that antagonised the effects of amphetamine and the doses needed to produce clinically effective changes[21]. This established that the D_2 receptor was an important site of action for the majority of antipsychotic agents. For some, this demonstration led on to a dopamine hypothesis of schizophrenia[16,24].

The dopamine hypothesis of schizophrenia in turn mandated an exclusive focus on the dopamine system and at least initially a focus on the D_2 receptor. New efforts were focused on producing D_2 receptor antagonists, in the belief that a selective D_2 receptor antagonist would be more effective and freer from side-effects. Through the 1980s this led to the synthesis of a series of compounds, culminating in the benzamide, remoxipride. Among the remaining drugs of this type on the market place are sulpiride and amisulpiride.

The relative failure of this approach to solve schizophrenia led some but not all to the abandonment of the dopamine hypothesis of schizophrenia. The emergence of D_3 and subsequently D_4 receptors meant that it remained possible to continue believing that some magical property of some yet to be discovered dopamine receptor would save this line of thinking[8]. This approach underpins ongoing efforts to test D_4 antagonists in schizophrenia.

From 1980, however, it had also become possible to radio-label serotonergic receptors[18]. Two $5HT_2$ antagonists, ritanserin and ketanserin, had already been developed by Janssen on the basis of an antagonism of the effects of tryptamines in animal models. Early clinical trials with these agents did not suggest that they would be effective stand-alone agents in the treatment of psychoses. But what about the combination of D_2–S_2 antagonists? The new receptor binding techniques made it possible to generate large series of new agents with this profile. This led to the synthesis of risperidone, a D_2 and S_2 antagonist. This turned out to be similar in many respects to the earlier dipiperone, except for potency[12]. Where doses in the order of 200–300 mg of dipiperone were needed clinically, doses of 2–3 mg of risperidone achieved the same effect in both binding assays and clinical practice. A similar approach led to the synthesis of sertindole[19]. The emergence of these agents and the re-emergence of clozapine led to debates about the relative merits of serotonergic and dopamine system antagonists (SDAs)[15].

This development has a rationality to it. However, it has involved a focussing down from the multiplicity of actions the original antipsychotics had, to an exclusive focus on selected monoamine receptor subtypes. It is quite possible that there are effects stemming from the 'dirtiness' of the original compounds that cannot be readily predicted from an analysis of the functional effects mediated by individual receptors[9]. Carlsson's more recent work points toward this possibility[2]. Another possibility is that hitherto ignored effects such as the original antihistaminic actions of these drugs may offer important therapeutic principles in a number of clinical cases[33].

Tardive dyskinesia

In the late 80s, clozapine re-emerged. The primary driving force behind its re-emergence was the fact that it was clear that this drug did not cause tardive dyskinesia. Concerns about the legal consequences of tardive dyskinesia had all but led to a suspension of antipsychotic drug development during the late 1970s and early 80s as the dimensions of this problem became clear[14,25]. Even before clozapine's re-introduction, the tardive dyskinesia problem had led to efforts on the part of major pharmaceutical companies to produce a tardive-dyskinesia-free antipsychotic.

There were a number of methods of so doing. One was to produce a structural analogue of clozapine. Essentially this is what olanzapine and quetiapine are. These agents were not developed on the basis of their receptor profile. In the case of quetiapine, in particular, an animal model of dyskinesia – the sensitised Cebus monkey model was used. The resulting receptor profile of quetiapine is a matter of interest but was not the driving force behind the production of the drug[34]. In fact, it is clear that there are a number of clozapine analogues that have closely related structural formulae and receptor profiles, which nevertheless produce dyskinesias. Olanzapine is one. It is not clear yet what, if anything, there is about the profile of action of these drugs on monoamine receptors that would explain the differences between these drugs in their propensity to cause dyskinesia.

In contrast, risperidone and sertindole were developed on the basis of their receptor profiles. These drugs, and coincidentally quetiapine and olanzapine, have a receptor profile that approximates more closely to that of earlier drugs such as chlorpromazine and chlorprothixene rather than later drugs such as haloperidol. It seems clear in terms of overall quality of life that this receptor profile is better suited to many patients than the receptor profile that results from efforts to antagonise the amphetamines. But some of the earlier agents with this profile, such as chlorpromazine and thioridazine, were nevertheless liable to produce tardive dyskinesia.

Two things can be pointed out about these developments. First, drugs based on amphetamine antagonising behavioural tests are not the same thing as drugs which have been synthesised as pure D_2 receptor blockers. The side-effect profile of sulpiride and amisulpiride, which are relatively specific D_2 receptor antagonists, is quite different to that of haloperidol or droperidol, which antagonise amphetamine effectively. Second, the additional actions on 5HT receptors may improve mental states by improving the quality of slow wave sleep, or by ameliorating some of the parkinsonism-inducing effects of amphetamine antagonists or by otherwise being personality strengthening, anxiolytic or antidepressant in some sense. They may also in some other, not-yet-determined, sense be antipsychotic. But the example of sulpiride and amisulpiride suggests that these effects are not a *sine qua non* for either antipsychotic activity or quality of life.

While in recent years the main focus has been on the additional benefits that $5HT_2$ (S_2) receptor antagonism may produce, it seems clear that in the cocktail of monoamine receptor actions an action on noradrenergic systems is also useful. There is convincing evidence from the early 1980s that noradrenergic re-uptake inhibitors, for example, can minimise the propensity of antipsychotics to cause extrapyramidal side-effects[29]. This explains why in some instances increasing the dose of haloperidol to the intermediate dose range (10–30 mg) may lead to marked extra pyramidal side-effects but increasing it further to 60 mg or more may lead to the disappearance of these effects. At these doses noradrenergic actions of the drug kick in. The addition of clonidine to standard neuroleptic regimes has appeared in some cases to produce clozapine-like effects[17,31].

It is clear that quite aside from their actions on monoamine receptors, the antipsychotics have a range of actions to block calcium channels of various types as well as other ion channels. This area of antipsychotic pharmacology remains unexplored. It may well be that their propensity to cause tardive dyskinesia or alternatively the quality which minimises that risk stems from an action of this sort. There is some evidence for this[30]. This point may relate to another area of antipsychotic pharmacology which remains unexplored – the differential propensity of these agents to produce discontinuation syndromes[10].

Positive and negative

The modern antipsychotics have not been sold on the back of their benefits for tardive dyskinesia however. They have been sold as agents, which are beneficial for the negative features of schizophrenia in the way that older agents supposedly were not. It should be noted, however, that this is not what they were developed for. There is in fact little evidence that they have the superior actions in this area claimed for them.

There is compelling data that older drugs, such as chlorpromazine, were beneficial for negative features of the illness and indeed more so for these features than for the supposed positive features of the illness[7]. The main difference between the prescribing of new and old drugs lies in the lower dose regimes that are used now compared with before. Owing to a risk of provoking epileptic convulsions, it was never possible to prescribe clozapine in doses that would give rise to marked extrapyramidal symptoms. It was, therefore, not possible to poison people with clozapine in the same ways that could be done with other agents. Prescribing newer agents in the dose regimes that are comparable to the clozapine doses means effectively a return to the kinds of doses and effects produced by lower dose chlorpromazine regimes from the mid-1950s through to the mid-1960s. No new agent has been shown to do better for negative symptoms than chlorpromazine prescribed in these doses. All comparisons of newer agents have been conducted with haloperidol in doses all but designed to produce drug-induced negative states.

There is at present no evidence that either clozapine or other newer antipsychotics are superior to conventional antipsychotics used in reasonable doses across a newly recruited sample of psychotic patients. The benefits of clozapine demonstrated in treatment resistance in Study 30[13] were benefits in a haloperidol-resistant population. The converse study, using haloperidol or other potent or selective D_2 antagonists in a clozapine-resistant population, remains to be undertaken and in fact a number of centres on an empirical basis are using drugs like amisulpiride as adjunctive agents in clozapine-resistant patients.

In contrast, in 1963 Fish reported[6] on the response rates of different types of schizophrenia to neuroleptics. He demonstrated an 85% response rate in certain paranoid states, falling to a 23% response rate for hebephrenia and a 1% response rate for systematic catatonia. There are no studies to indicate that these poorly responsive schizophrenic subtypes preferentially respond to any agents, which have emerged from the mid-1960s onwards. This suggests that the real residual therapeutic problems post-chlorpromazine remain effectively untouched. There have perhaps been more advances in the area of market slogans than there have been in the area of real therapeutic advances, at least where severe schizophrenic syndromes are concerned. The only significant development has been in so far as there has been an optimisation of the ability to avoid tardive dyskinesia.

Coda

For twenty years following the development of the antipsychotics, there was a major disjunction between the theories of what was wrong in psychoses and theories about how the drugs acted. Earlier theories such as the transmethylation hypotheses kept open the possibility of alternate therapeutic interventions in a way that later dopamine related hypotheses have not done. Equally, during the first twenty years, antipsychotic drug development was driven by efforts to 'optimise' various properties of the drug in a manner that was not hidebound by theories of what was supposedly wrong in the illness.

More recently, there has been a conjunction of psychopathophysiological theories and drug development models that has reduced antipsychotic drug development to increasing sterility. The scope for thinking outside a narrow confine has become greatly limited. The field awaits another unexpected albeit rational development – another chlorpromazine.

References

1. Carlsson A, Lindqvist M (1963). Effect of chlorpromazine or haloperidol on the formation of

3-methoxytyramine and normetanephrine in mouse brain. *Acta Pharmacol* (Kbh) 20, 140–144.
2. Carlsson A, Carlsson M (1994). Interactions between glutamatergic and monoaminergic systems within the basal ganglia – implications for schizophrenia and Parkinson's disease. *Trends Neursci* 13, 272–276.
3. Comite Lyonnais de Recherches Therapeutiques en Psychiatrie (2000). The Birth of Psychopharmacotherapy: Explorations in a New World 1952–1968. In Healy D. *The Psychopharmacologists* vol. 3, Arnold, London, pp. 1–53.
4. Creese I, Burt DR, Snyder S (1976). Dopamine receptor binding predicts clinical and pharmacological potencies of antischizophrenic drugs. *Science* 192, 481–483.
5. Delay J, Deniker P, Harl JM (1952). Utilisation en thérapeutique psychiatrique d'une phénothiazine d'action centrale élective. *Ann Méd Psychol* 110, 112–117.
6. Fish FJ (1963). The influence of the tranquillizers on the Leonhard schizophrenic syndromes. *Encephale* 53, 245–249.
7. Goldberg S, Cole JO, Klerman GL (1964). Phenothiazine treatment in acute schizophenia. *Archives of General Psychiatry* 10, 246–261.
8. Healy D (1991). D-1, D-2 and D-3. *British J Psychiatry* 159, 319–324.
9. Healy D (1999). Antidepressant psychopharmacotherapy at the crossroads. *Int J Psychiatry in Clin Practice* 3 (supp. 2), S9–S15.
10. Healy D, Tranter R (1999). Pharmacopsychiatric stress diathesis syndromes. *J Psychopharmacology* 13, 287–299.
11. Healy D (2002). *The Creation of Psychopharmacology*. Harvard University Press, Cambridge Mass.
12. Janssen P (1998). From haloperidol to risperidone. In Healy D, *The Psychopharmacologists* vol. 2, pp. 39–70, Chapman & Hall, London.
13. Kane J, Honigfeld G, Singer J, Meltzer H (1988). Clozapine for the treatment-resistant schizophenic. *Archives of General Psychiatry* 45, 789–796.
14. Lieberman JA, Saltz BL, Johns CA, Pollack S, Borenstein M, Kane J (1991). The effects of clozapine on tardive dyskinesia. *British J Psychaitry* 158, 503–510.
15. Meltzer HY (1992). The mechanism of action of novel antipsychotic drugs. *Schizophrenia Bulletin* 17, 263–287.
16. Meltzer HY, Stahl S (1976). The dopamine hypothesis of schizophrenia: a review. *Schizophrenia Bulletin* 2, 19–76.
17. Nutt D (1994). Putting the A in atypical: does alpha2-adrenoceptor antagonism account for the therapeutic advantage of new antipsychotics? *J Psychopharmacology* 8, 193–195.
18. Peroutka S, Snyder SH (1979). Multiple serotonin receptors: differential binding of 3H.5-hydroxytryptamine, 3H.lysergic acid diethylamide and 3H.spiroperidol. *Molecular Pharmacology* 16, 687–699.
19. Pedersen V, Bogeso K. (1998). Drug Hunting. In Healy D, *The Psychopharmacologists* vol. 2, Chapman & Hall, London, pp. 561–579.
20. Schmutz and Eichenberger Schmutz J, Eichenberger E (1982). Clozapine. *Chronicles of Drug Discovery* 1, 39–59.
21. Seeman P, Lee T, Chau-Wong M, Wong K (1976). Antipsychotic drug doses and neuroleptic/dopamine receptors. *Nature* 261, 717–719.
22. Snyder S (2000). Visualising receptors and beyond. In Healy D, *The Psychopharmacologists* vol. 3, Arnold, London.
23. Snyder S, Banerjee SP, Yamamora HI, Greenberg A (1974). Drugs, neurotoxins and schizophrenia. *Science* 188, 1243–1245.
24. Snyder S (1976). The dopamine hypothesis of schizophrenia; focus on the dopamine receptor. *American J Psychiatry* 133, 197–202.
25. Sugarman AA (2000). Remembrance of drugs past. In Ban T, Healy D, Shorter E (eds), *The Triumph of Psychopharmacology*, Animula, Budapest.
26. Sugarman AA (1964). A pilot study of fluoropipamide (Dipiperone). *Diseases of the Nervous System* 25, 355–358.
27. Swazey J (1974). *Chlorpromazine. A Study in Therapeutic Innovation*. MIT Press, Cambridge, Mass.
28. Thuillier (1980/1999). *Les Dix Ans qui on Changé la Folie*, translated as 'Ten Years Which Changed The Face Of Mental Illness'. Hickish G, Healy D. Martin Dunitz & Co., London.
29. Toru M (1981). Haloperidol in large doses reduces the cataleptic response and increases noradrenaline metabolism in the brain of the rat. *Neuropharmacology* 24, 231–236.
30. Tranter R, Healy D (1998). Neuroleptic discontinuation syndromes. *J Psychopharmacology* 12, 401–406.
31. Van Kammen D P, Gelernter J (1987). The biochemical instability in schizophrenia 1: the norepinephrine system. *Psychopharmacology: The Third Generation of Progress*, Meltzer H, Raven Press, New York, pp. 745–751.
32. Van Rossum (1966). The significance of dopamine receptor blockade in the mechanism of

action of neuroleptic drugs. *Archives of International Pharmacodynamics & Therapeutics* 60, 492–494.

33. Vinar O (2000). A Psychopharamacology that Nearly Was. In Healy D, *The Psychopharmacologists* vol. 3, Arnold, London, pp. 55–79.

34. Warawa E (2000). From neuroleptics to antipsychotics. In Healy D, *The Psychopharmacologists* vol. 3, Arnold, pp. 505–524.

Chapter 3

ECT: an Effective, but Ignored, Treatment of Psychosis*

Professor Max Fink

Introduction

Communities throughout the nation bear large numbers of the chronic mentally ill in our prisons, in isolated and impersonal half-way houses, and in shelters for the homeless. They once resided in state mental hospitals, but a precipitous down-sizing has thrown them onto the community's streets to become major actors in our revolving-door hospital admissions. For these patients, one antipsychotic medicine after another is prescribed in a complex polypharmacy, with instructions that our patients follow poorly.

Can more be done? Do we have more knowledge that we can apply? An answer lies in electroconvulsive therapy, a treatment that often benefits these patients, but one that is hardly available at the treatment venues that these patients attend[26]. ECT has such a bad name that even clinicians who are skilled in its use prefer to offer their patients less effective but less criticized options. Personal and public bias, lack of training among psychiatrists, and legislative and judicial proscriptions are additional hurdles. This essay summarizes our knowledge of ECT in the treatment of psychosis and urges a re-assessment of its role in our therapy programs.

In the second quarter of the 20th century, the principal treatments for psychotic patients were insulin coma, leucotomy, and electroconvulsive therapy. The discovery of the antipsychotic effects of reserpine and chlorpromazine challenged their use.

For insulin coma, a random assignment comparison found chlorpromazine to be effective, safe, and less expensive[27]. It was not that chlorpromazine was a markedly better treatment, for the clinical efficacy of the two treatments was comparable, but insulin coma's morbidity and mortality and the medications' ease of use led to the rapid closure of insulin treatment units.

For leucotomy, no direct comparison with antipsychotic drugs was made but the success rate of surgery had been so low, the side-effects so severe, and its acceptance so poor that the new drugs ended clinical interest. Psychosurgery remains in occasional use for experimental purposes.

For ECT, the comparisons with antipsychotic drugs found both treatments to be similarly effective[1,18,26]. The risks of the new drugs were not yet known, so the immediate ill effects of ECT in inducing fractures, confusion, and memory deficits tipped the clinical balance in favor of the drugs. The ease of administration and their assumed greater safety, not a superior efficacy, favored the use of the medicines over ECT.

While the new medicines suppress symptoms, few patients recover fully. Prolonged use brings on the risks of tardive dyskinesia, parkinsonism, and dystonia. Sudden deaths occur. When these deaths were better understood as examples of the neuroleptic malignant syndrome, treatments were developed, and the mortality rate of 25% before 1984 was reduced to 12% by 1989, a not so trivial risk[51,68]. For many patients, however, neither the new drugs or more effective surrogates nor diverse augmentation strategies have measurably reduced the widespread problem of pharmacotherapy-resistant psychosis[31,37].

The marketing of clozapine in the 1990s, a drug with a history of toxicity that had led to its

---

*Convulsive Therapy in Schizophrenia? By Fink M, Sackeim HA (*Schizophrenia Bulletin* 1996; 22:27–39) contains an extensive review of the studies of ECT and antipsychotic drugs, and is the background for this essay.

recall a decade earlier, is an example of the public willingness to use a medicine despite a considerable known risk and a limited efficacy. The first reports showed clozapine to reduce psychosis rating scale scores by 30% in 30% of the patients[42]. Despite its potential toxicity, this small benefit was sufficient to encourage the acceptance of its use and for the public to demand state governments to make clozapine widely available. Clozapine was labeled an 'atypical neuroleptic' and international pharmaceutical companies spent millions of dollars to find substances with similar pharmacologic profiles, leading to the marketing of risperidone, olanzapine, and quetiapine. These drugs have been useful, but have hardly relieved the problem of pharmacotherapy resistance.

The desire for a more effective and safer antipsychotic treatment led to a re-examination of the experience with ECT[1,3]. Professional attitudes were confused. Those physicians who had treated acutely ill schizophrenic patients recalled ECT as effective, noting however that the patients required many more treatments than did their depressed or manic patients. Those physicians who treated the chronically ill, especially those patients that had been warehoused in state facilities for prolonged periods, recalled much poorer results. Since more chronic patients than acutely ill had been treated with ECT, the belief was widely held that ECT was ineffective in treating schizophrenia, justifying its rejection[3,18].

A literature review of 60 years of experience with ECT in schizophrenia found:

"... it [ECT] to be an effective treatment for psychosis. ECT is particularly applicable in patients with first-break episodes, especially those marked by excitement, overactivity, delusions, or delirium; in the young to avoid the debilitating effects of chronic illness; and in syndromes characterized by catatonia, 'positive symptoms of psychosis', or schizoaffective features."[26]

The authors argued:

"... for the use of ECT early in the course of treatment of acutely psychotic patients, especially in first-break psychotic patients with excitement, overactivity, delusions, or florid delirium, and in those who are young, to avoid the debilitating effects of chronic illness. If patients are treated effectively early in the course of their illness, we believe that the risks of chronicity of illness and deterioration in personality can be avoided."

Recognizing that the first line use of ECT in schizophrenia would be difficult to justify on the available evidence, the authors recommended:

"There is need for prospective studies of ECT alone or ECT combined with neuroleptic drugs contrasted with neuroleptic drugs alone in patients with schizophrenia. Since the efficacy of combined medication and ECT is probably greater than ECT alone, combined therapy should be favored in prospective assessments."

The consideration of ECT in psychotic patients comes after they have failed multiple medication trials and complex combinations. Referral for ECT is as the last recourse, when the patients and families ask whether the physicians can recommend anything other than another medication trial, or when the patients become so aggressive and agitated as to force hospital admission and the search for a more effective treatment. Professional concerns about the recurrence of psychosis and worsening of dyskinesia when antipsychotic drugs are discontinued makes it common practice for prescribed medicines, even in complex combinations, to be continued when ECT is added.

ECT as augmentation

Recent reports find the augmentation of ongoing antipsychotic medications by ECT to elicit improvement and, on occasion, even recovery from the illness. The successful augmentation by ECT of failed thiothixene treatment in nine medication-resistant psychotic patients was first reported by Friedel[30]. His report encouraged a retrospective review in eight schizophrenic patients who had not improved with medication alone and had received ECT. Seven had successful outcomes[34]. When loxapine was augmented by ECT, measures of psychosis improved[67]. But the experience with clozapine and ECT that provides compelling evidence of the merit of ECT augmentation.

The augmentation of clozapine by ECT was recognized by two reporters who described the response of their patients as 'remarkable'[44,45,50]. Additional clinical examples quickly dotted the literature[6,7,8,11,12,13,15,17,28,33,38,39,41,48,53,62,66]. Delusional thought, aggressivity, hallucinations, apathy, and withdrawal show the most relief. In a prospective study in progress, Petrides and Mendelowitz[62] reported a greater than 40% reduction in BPRS psychosis scores in 7/12 patients who had failed multiple medication trials, including high doses of clozapine for extended durations. These pilot studies encouraged the NIMH (National Institute of Mental Health) to support a prospective controlled study in which clozapine-resistant psychotic patients are randomly assigned to continued clozapine or to ECT augmentation of continued clozapine, each for a minimum of eight weeks.

The interest in ECT augmentation of clozapine should not detract from the use of ECT with any antipsychotic medicine. Such synergy is well documented[19–21,23–4,26,46].

ECT compared to drugs in psychoses other than schizophrenia

Psychotic patients are commonly first treated with antipsychotic drugs. But for those with psychotic depression and delirious mania, two well-defined psychoses, the efficacy of antipsychotic drugs alone is poor. The concept of psychotic depression owes its recognition to the studies of Glassman and his associates who were monitoring imipramine treatment with weekly serum levels in hospitalized depressed patients[32,43]. Despite adequate imipramine serum levels, only three of 13 psychotic depressed patients (30%) improved compared to 14 of 21 non-psychotic depressed patients (66%). Nine of the 10 unimproved psychotic depressed patients recovered with subsequent ECT. They concluded that the treatment of psychotic depressed patients with only a tricyclic antidepressant prolonged the suffering, increased the risk for suicide, and unnecessarily exposed them to toxicity.

This report was quickly confirmed. Italian investigators treated 437 depressed hospitalized patients with imipramine in doses of 200 to 350 mg/day for 25 days or longer[5]. Of these, 247 patients (57%) recovered and were discharged. Each of the 190 unimproved patients was next treated with bilateral ECT, and of these, 156 (72%) recovered. Of the depressed patients who had not improved with imipramine, 43% were also psychotic.

By 1985, Kroessler summarized reports that found that half the psychotic depressed patients recovered when treated with antipsychotic drugs alone, and even fewer, approximately a third, improved with antidepressant drugs alone. With both antipsychotic and tricyclic antidepressant drugs together, or with ECT, two-thirds improved. Two recent reviews confirm this assessment: Parker et al.[61] and Vega et al.[73].

Delirious mania is a psychotic syndrome of the acute onset of delusions, excitement, grandiosity, emotional lability, and insomnia characteristic of mania, and the disorientation and altered consciousness characteristic of delirium[23–4]. Psychoactive drug toxicity, systemic illness, mania, and depression are common antecedents. Catatonia is a frequent accompaniment, and it is difficult to distinguish delirious mania from excited or malignant catatonia. Delirious mania is usually treated with antipsychotic drugs but such use is associated with neurotoxic risks. The most effective and safest alternative is ECT.

In patients with psychotic depression and delirious mania, ECT provides effective antipsychotic actions when used alone, and is more effective than antipsychotic drugs.

Adverse events, contraindications, and interactions

The combination of antipsychotic drugs and ECT is remarkably safe[1,4,46,58]. Indeed, for tardive dyskinesia, parkinsonism, and neuroleptic malignant syndrome, ECT reduces the severity of these motor syndromes.

ECT does not worsen psychosis. Its benefits require many treatments so that the immediate confusional effects of each treatment may become prominent. But when the psychosis resolves and continuation treatments are spaced further apart in time, confusion wanes and the relief of psychosis becomes the dominant experience.

Also for the combined use of clozapine and ECT, adverse effects are remarkably few. In a single case, Beale et al.[6] reported that the administration of caffeine to achieve a longer seizure with ECT in a patient receiving clozapine elicited a prolonged period of supraventricular tachycardia. Other than this experience, the literature is mute with regard to adverse effects of ECT augmented clozapine treatment.

Mode of action

How are we to understand the synergism of antipsychotic drugs and ECT? Two aspects of physiology are relevant. Antipsychotic drugs lower seizure thresholds and spontaneous seizures have been reported for many antipsychotic drugs, especially chlorpromazine and clozapine[46]. At high doses, clozapine (and other atypical antipsychotic drugs) elicit EEG seizure activity in both humans and in animals. Evoked grand-mal seizures are occasionally reported[16, 35, 36, 40, 41, 52, 54, 57, 63, 69, 75]. An association between the degree of EEG slowing and serum clozapine levels is reported[29,59]. These observations led Stevens[71] to explain the beneficial effects of clozapine as due to increased excitability in subcortical brain areas, an idea that is consistent with concepts of the antagonism of seizures and psychosis[56,72].

The paradoxical association between behavioral improvement in emotional disorders with the development of EEG epileptic rhythms was discussed in studies of epileptic psychotic patients[49]. When epileptic patients were treated with anticonvulsant drugs, so that their EEG records normalized and their seizures were controlled, they exhibited psychotic symptoms. When the medication dosages were reduced, seizures and EEG abnormalities returned, and their clinical behavior improved. This association has been labeled 'forced normalization' or 'paradoxical normalization'[60,72,74]. (It was the apparent antagonism between epileptic seizures and the psychotic symptoms of dementia praecox that led Meduna to envision and develop convulsive therapy for the relief of dementia praecox[56]).

During ECT, the inter-seizure EEG is progressively filled with slow wave activity and seizure-like bursts. The development and persistence of EEG slowing and burst activity is related to the clinical outcome[18,25,64,65]. Patients who fail to develop high degrees of EEG slowing fail to improve clinically.

Indeed, the development of an abnormal EEG (slowing of frequencies, development of burst activity) during clozapine therapy is associated with a better clinical outcome compared to the results when the EEG fails to change[63].

A second item of physiology that helps us understand the benefit of ECT augmentation is a seizure-induced greater penetrability of the blood-brain-barrier (BBB). The BBB ordinarily prevents large chemical molecules from crossing into the CNS from the vascular compartment. ECT increases the permeability of the BBB, allowing large molecules to cross into the CNS[2,9,10]. While the effect on the BBB of a single seizure is of short duration, repeated seizures allow the persistent transport of materials. The penetration of substances varies in different brain regions[14]. We envision greater amounts of clozapine entering the brain without the systemic problems incurred when high tissue levels are developed in other body systems.

These two physiologic factors explain the benefit of ECT augmentation of clozapine therapy. Both ECT and clozapine induce EEG seizure activity, a change that is operationally associated with a reduction in psychosis. The clinical efficacy of clozapine is dose-related, with higher doses having greater benefits. But high doses of clozapine are associated with systemic drowsiness, sialorrhea, and seizures, limiting the upper dosing levels. The ECT related changes in the BBB allows greater amounts of clozapine to pass to the brain without adverse systemic effects, encouraging a more robust CNS effect of clozapine. The same benefit accrues to the augmentation of other antipsychotic drugs by ECT.

Treatment algorithms and ECT

Modern medical practice increasingly asks for evidence-based treatment decisions. The decisions are codified in algorithms produced by assembled 'experts'. As we lack robust experimental studies of the efficacy of the new antipsychotic drugs, either alone or compared to ECT, the expert recommendations are based, almost exclusively and of necessity, on testimonials. Few experts treat many patients personally (most manage data collecting networks of treating doctors and nurses), and fewer still have experience with ECT. As a consequence,

ECT is hardly considered in their algorithms; when it is considered, it is as the last resort in the algorithm, or listed in a footnote among miscellaneous treatments.

This attitude is both inhumane and uneconomic. It is inhumane because it fails to use an effective and safe treatment in a timely fashion. Patients with resolvable illnesses remain unwell and unproductive for themselves, their families, and society. It is uneconomic since the overall cost of a course of ECT is often less than repeated courses of medications especially when lost wages are factored into the estimates[55,70].

A more reasonable guideline for the use of ECT in treating psychosis comes from the standard used to evaluate clozapine when it was known to be severely toxic. To assure that only treatment refractory patients were subjected to the possible toxicity of clozapine, the committees supporting such research argued that patients would have to fail two medication trials with antipsychotic drugs of two different classes, at adequate clinical dosages, each for a minimum of six weeks. Failure to improve with treatments of this rigorous standard justified exposure to the potentially toxic alternative[42]. Since that model was successful in marketing clozapine, it is reasonable to apply the same standard to the decision to use ECT in treating psychosis. Instead of interminable trials of antipsychotic drugs, psychotic patients should be referred for ECT augmentation after two antipsychotic medication trials have failed, or earlier in those patients who are suicidal, suffering from inanition, catatonia, or are medically ill.

Conclusion

The efficacy of ECT in relieving psychosis is a clinical benefit that is infrequently recognized. When ECT was replaced by antipsychotic drugs, it was not that the drugs were more effective or even safer. The replacement was for the ease of use of the medicines, their widespread availability, and the antipathy to the use of ECT. In the four decades since the introduction of antipsychotic drugs, we have become inured to their side-effects. We tolerate tardive dyskinesia, neuroleptic malignant syndrome, parkinsonism, akathisia, unexplained deaths, and the development of apathy, withdrawal, and loss of motivation that characterizes the secondary effects of their prolonged use. At the same time, the risks of ECT in fracture, death, and cognitive impairment that at one time characterized the side-effects of ECT have been materially reduced. Indeed, there is no medical illness or physical condition that precludes the use of ECT when the psychiatric indications call for its use.

The apathy of the profession results in ECT being ignored in the spate of treatment algorithms that are now being written. As these algorithms become codified in the management of the severe mentally ill, the benefits of ECT will become even more difficult to achieve. Our multi-tier system of mental health care, in which the insured are able to obtain care in private and university psychiatric services (where ECT is available) while the indigent depend on state supported facilities (where ECT is not available), further disadvantages the mentally ill poor and the minorities of all nations. Such failure consigns many hundreds, if not thousands, of patients to the prolonged misery of the positive and negative symptoms of schizophrenia, the loss of their most productive years in work, and their isolation from friends and family. The antipathy and apathy among psychiatrists and other mental health professionals toward an effective treatment is a sad commentary on the present education of psychiatrists and their co-workers. As our education is increasingly dominated by a pharmaceutical industry that ignores competing therapies, it becomes likely that few of the next generation of mental health workers will have experience with ECT. While the pre-eminence of the use of medications for psychotic patients is explained by their ease of use and efficacy, ECT augmentation of antipsychotic drugs compels greater attention to this combination for the relief of the burdens of pharmacotherapy-resistant psychosis.

References

1. Abrams R. *Electroconvulsive Therapy*. Oxford University Press, NY, 3rd edition, 1997, 382 pp.
2. Aird RB, Strait I. Protective barriers of the central nervous system: An experimental study with trypan red. *Arch Neurol Psychiatry* 1945; 51:54–66.

3. American Psychiatric Association. *Electroconvulsive Therapy. Task Force Report.* American Psychiatric Association, Washington DC, 1978.
4. American Psychiatric Association. *Electroconvulsive Therapy: Recommendations for Treatment, Training and Privileging.* American Psychiatric Association, Washington DC, 1990.
5. Avery D, Lubrano A. Depression treated with imipramine and ECT: the deCarolis study reconsidered. *Am J Psychiatry* 1979; 136:559–62.
6. Beale MD, Pritchett JT, Kellner, CH. Supraventricular tachycardia in a patient receiving ECT, clozapine, and caffeine. *Convulsive Ther.* 1994; 10:228–31.
7. Benatov R, Sirota P, Megged S. Neuroleptic-resistant schizophrenia treated with clozapine and ECT. *Convulsive Ther* 1996; 12:117–21.
8. Bhatia SC, Bhatia SK, Gupta S. Concurrent administration of clozapine and ECT: a successful therapeutic strategy for a patient with treatment-resistant schizophrenia. *JECT* 1998; 14: 280–283.
9. Bolwig T, Hertz MM, Holm-Jensen J. Blood–brain barrier permeability during electroshock seizures in the rat. *Eur J Clin Invest* 1977a; 7:95–100.
10. Bolwig T, Hertz MM, Paulson OB *et al.* The permeability of the blood–brain barrier during electrically induced seizures in man. *Eur J Clin Invest* 1977b; 7:87–93.
11. Cardwell BA, Nakai B. Seizure activity in combined clozapine and ECT: a retrospective view. *Convulsive Ther.* 1995; 11:110–3.
12. Chanpattana W. Combined ECT and clozapine in treatment-resistant mania. *JECT* 2000; 16: 204–207.
13. Chanpattana W, Chakrabhand S, Kongsakon R *et al.* The short-term effect of combined ECT and neuroleptic therapy in therapy-resistant schizophrenia. *JECT* 1999; 15:129–139.
14. Cutler RWP, Lorenzo AV, Barlow CF. Changes in blood–brain permeability during pharmacologically induced convulsions. *Prog Brain Research* 1968; 29:367–378.
15. Dassa D, Kaladjian A, Azorin JM, Giudicelli S. Clozapine in the treatment of psychotic refractory depression. *Br J Psychiatry* 1993; 163:822–4.
16. Denney D, Stevens JR. Clozapine and seizures. *Biol Psychiatry* 1995; 37:427–33.
17. Factor SA, Molho ES, Brown DL. Combined clozapine and electroconvulsive therapy for the treatment of drug-induced psychosis in Parkinson's Disease. *J Neuropsychiatry Clin Neurosci.* 1995; 7:304–7.
18. Fink M. *Convulsive therapy: Theory and practice.* Raven Press, New York 1979, 306 pp.
19. Fink M. Clozapine and electroconvulsive therapy. *Arch Gen Psychiatry* 1990; 47:290–1 (Letter).
20. Fink M. Pharmacotherapy and ECT. *Convulsive Ther* 1991; 7:77–80.
21. Fink M. ECT and clozapine in schizophrenia. *JECT* 1998; 14:223–26.
22. Fink, M. The decision to use ECT: For Whom? When? In: AJ Rush [Ed]: *Mood Disorders: Systematic Medication Management. Modern Probl. Pharmacopsychiatry.* 1997; 25:203–14. Karger, Basel, Switzerland.
23. Fink M. *Electroshock: Restoring the Mind,* Oxford University Press, New York, 1999a, 157 pp.
24. Fink M. Delirious mania. *Bipolar Disorders* 1999b; 1:54–60.
25. Fink M, Kahn RL. Relation of EEG delta activity to behavioral response to electroshock: Quantitative serial studies. *Arch Gen Psychiatry* 1957; 39:1189–91.
26. Fink M, Sackeim HA. Convulsive therapy in schizophrenia? *Schiz Bull* 1996; 22:27–39.
27. Fink M, Shaw R, Gross G, Coleman FS. Comparative study of chlorpromazine and insulin coma in the therapy of psychosis. *JAMA* 1958b; 166:1846–50.
28. Frankenburg FR, Suppes T, McLean PE. Combined clozapine and electroconvulsive therapy. *Convulsive Ther.* 1993; 9:176–80.
29. Freudenreich O, Weiner RD, McEvoy JP. Clozapine-induced electroencephalogram changes as a function of clozapine serum levels. *Biol Psychiatry* 1997; 42:132–7.
30. Friedel RO. The combined use of neuroleptics and ECT in drug resistant schizophrenic patients. *Psychopharmacol Bull* 1986; 22:928–30.
31. Gelman S. *Medicating Schizophrenia.* New Brunswick NJ: Rutgers University Press, 1999, 274 pp.
32. Glassman AH, Kantor SJ, Shostak M. Depression, delusions, and drug response. *Am J Psychiatry* 1975; 132:716–9. The delusional depressed patients responded to courses of ECT.
33. Green AI, Zalma A, Berman I, *et al.*, Clozapine following ECT: a two-step treatment. *J Clin Psychiatry* 1994; 55(9):388–90.
34. Gujavarty K, Greenberg L, Fink M. Electroconvulsive therapy and neuroleptic medication in therapy-resistant positive symptom psychosis. *Convulsive Ther* 1987; 3:185–95.
35. Gunther W, Baghai T, Naber D *et al.* EEG alterations and seizures during treatment with cloz-

35. apine. A retrospective study of 283 patients. *Pharmacopsychiatry* 1993; 26:69–74.
36. Haring C, Neudorfer C, Schwitzer J et al. EEG alterations in patients treated with clozapine in relation to plasma levels. *Psychopharmacol* 1994; 114:97–110.
37. Healy D. *The Creation of Psychopharmacology*. Boston: Harvard University Press, (in press).
38. Hirose S, Ashby CR, Mills MJ. Effectiveness of ECT combined with risperidone against aggression in schizophrenia. JECT 2001; 17:22–6.
39. James DV, Gray NS. Elective combined electroconvulsive and clozapine therapy. *Internat Clin Psychopharmacology* 1999; 14:69–72.
40. Jin Y, Potkin SG, Sandman C. Clozapine increases EEG photic driving in clinical responders. *Schiz Bull* 1995; 21:263–268.
41. Kales HC, DeQuardo JR, Tandon R. Combined electroconvulsive therapy and clozapine in treatment-resistant schizophrenia. *Prog Neuro-Psychopharm Biol Psychiatry* 1999; 23:547–556.
42. Kane J, Honingfeld G, Singer J, et al. Clozapine for the treatment-resistant schizophrenic: a double-blind comparison with chlorpromazine. *Arch Gen Psychiatry* 1988; 45:789–796.
43. Kantor SJ, Glassman AH. Delusional depressions: natural history and response to treatment. *Br J Psychiatry* 1977; 131:351–60.
44. Klapheke MM. Clozapine, ECT, and schizoaffective disorder, bipolar type. *Convulsive Ther.* 1991a; 7:36–9.
45. Klapheke MM. Follow-up on clozapine and ECT. *Convulsive Ther.* 1991b; 7:303–5.
46. Klapheke MM. Combining ECT and antipsychotic agents: Benefits and risks. *Convulsive Ther* 1993; 9:241–55.
47. Kroessler D. Relative efficacy rates for therapies of delusional depression. *Convulsive Ther.* 1985; 1:173–82.
48. Kupchik M, Spivak B, Mester R et al. Combined electroconvulsive–clozapine therapy. *Clin Neuropharmacol* 2000; 23:14–16.
49. Landolt H. Serial electroencephalographic investigations during psychotic episodes in epileptic patients and during schizophrenic attacks. In: L de Haas (Ed.) *Lectures on Epilepsy*. Elsevier, NY, 1958; 3:91–133.
50. Landy DA. Combined use of clozapine and electroconvulsive therapy. *Convulsive Ther.* 1991;7: 218–21.
51. Lazarus A, Mann SC, Caroff SN. *The Neuroleptic Malignant Syndrome and Related Conditions*. Washington DC: American Psychiatric Press, Inc., 1989.
52. Lee JW, Crismon ML, Dorson PG. Seizure associated with olanzapine. *Ann Pharmacother* 1999; 33:554–6.
53. Lurie SN. Combined use of ECT and clozapine *J Clin Psychiatry* 1996; 57:94–5.
54. Malow BA, Reese KB, Sato et al. Spectrum of EEG abnormalities during clozapine treatment. *EEG clin Neurophysiol* 1994; 91:205–11.
55. Markowitz J, Brown R, Sweeney J, et al. Reduced length and cost of hospital stay for major depression in patients treated with ECT. *Am J Psychiatry* 1987; 144:1025–9.
56. Meduna L. Autobiography. *Convulsive Ther.* 1985; 1:43–57; 121–38.
57. Neufeld MY, Rabey JM, Orlov E, et al. Electroencephalographic findings of low-dose clozapine treatment in psychotic Parkinsonian patients. *Clin Neuropharm* 1996; 19:81–86.
58. Nobler MS, Sackeim HA. Augmentation strategies in electroconvulsive therapy: A synthesis. *Convulsive Ther.* 1993; 9:331–51.
59. Olesen OV, Thomsen K, Jensen PN et al. Clozapine serum levels and side effects during steady state treatment of schizophrenic patients: a cross sectional study. *Psychopharmacol* 1995; 117:371–378.
60. Pakalnis A, Drake ME, John K, et al. Forced normalization. Acute psychosis after seizure control in seven patients. *Arch Neurol* 1987; 44:289–92.
61. Parker G, Roy K, Hadzi-Pavlovic D. Psychotic (delusional) depression: A meta-analysis of physical treatments. *J Affective Dis* 1992; 24:17–24.
62. Petrides G, Mendelowitz A. Preliminary findings in ECT augmentation of clozapine in clozapine-resistant psychotic patients. Personal communication, September 2000.
63. Risby ED, Epstein CM, Jewart Rd et al. Clozapine-induced EEG abnormalities and clinical response to clozapine. *J Neurpsych clin Neurosci* 1995; 7:466–470.
64. Roth M. Changes in the EEG under barbiturate anesthesia produced by electro-convulsive treatment and their significance for the theory of ECT action. *Electroenceph clin Neurophysiol* 1951; 3:261–80.
65. Sackeim HA, Luber B, Katzman GP, et al. The effects of electroconvulsive therapy on quantitative electroencephalograms. *Arch gen Psychiatry* 1996; 53:814–824.
66. Safferman AZ, Munne R. Case report. Combining clozapine with ECT. *Convulsive Ther.* 1992; 8:141–3.

67. Sajatovic M, Meltzer HH. The effect of short-term electroconvulsive treatment plus neuroleptics in treatment-resistant schizophrenia and schizoaffective disorder. *Convulsive Ther* 1993; 9:167–75.
68. Shalev A, Hermesh H, Munitz H. Mortality from neuroleptic malignant syndrome. *J Clin Psychiatry* 1989; 50:18–25.
69. Silvestri RC, Bromfield EB, Khoshbin S. Clozapine-induced seizures and EEG abnormalities in ambulatory psychiatric patients. *Ann Pharmacother* 1998; 32:1147–51.
70. Steffens DC, Krystal AD, Sibert TE et al. Cost effectiveness of maintenance ECT. *Convulsive Ther.* 1995; 11:283–4.
71. Stevens JR. Clozapine: the Yin and Yang of seizures and psychosis *Biol Psychiatry* 1995;37: 425–6.
72. Trimble MR. Forced normalization and alternative psychoses. *The Psychoses of Epilepsy*, Raven Press, NY, 1991; 5:65–78.
73. Vega JAW, Mortimer AM, Tyson PJ. Somatic treatment of psychotic depression: Review and recommendations for practice. *Jrl Clinical Psychopharmacology* 2000; 20:504–19.
74. Wolf P, Trimble MR. Biological antagonism and epileptic psychosis. *Br J Psychiatry* 1985; 146: 272–6.
75. Wyderski RJ, Starrett WG, Abou-Saif A. Fatal status epilepticus associated with olanzapine therapy. *Ann Pharmacother* 1999; 33:787–9.

Chapter 4
Prediction of Response to Lithium in Affective Disorders

Dr M T Abou-Saleh

Introduction

The rediscovery of lithium and its reintroduction to psychiatry in 1949 has provided one of the most dramatic developments in psychiatric practice. Indeed it has antedated the introduction of chlorpromazine in 1957 and imipramine in 1962. Moreover its established efficacy in the management of manic depressive psychosis has affirmed Kraeplin's distinction between schizophrenia and manic depressive psychosis and later on the distinction between bipolar and unipolar affective disorder. Its efficacy in the management of affective disorders has been established by numerous high quality controlled studies which showed that the use of lithium substantially reduces the morbidity and mortality of recurrent affective disorders[12]. However, the impact of lithium on the naturalistic outcome of affective disorders was challenged by Dickson and Kendell[16] who reported a three-fold increase of admissions for mania to the Royal Edinburgh Hospital between 1970 and 1981, despite a ten-fold increase in the use of lithium during that period. Goodwin and Jamison[18] criticised the study referring to factors that could have contributed to this finding: diagnostic shift from schizophrenia to mania, the increased incidence of drug and alcohol misuse and the increased use of antidepressants resulting in greater risk for mania or lithium-resistant mania. Naturalistic studies reported from the Lithium Clinic in Epsom, however, consistently reported higher rates of efficacy for lithium in both bipolar and unipolar illness[5] including studies evaluating lower doses/levels of lithium[13]. Two recent Cochrane Systematic reviews have supported the use and usefulness of lithium in the maintenance treatment of mood disorders. The first review[10] indicated that lithium therapy compared to placebo is effective in the maintenance treatment of mood disorder, particularly bipolar disorders. The second review[25] of the efficacy of valproic acid, valproate and divalproex in the maintenance treatment of bipolar disorder reported that the evidence for their efficacy compared to placebo and lithium is inconclusive and advocated the use of lithium before valproate for maintenance treatment.

Lithium has also been shown to have antisuicidal effects in retrospective trials reducing mortality by 80% in patients with recurrent mood disorders[14]. Baldessarini et al.[9] in reviewing 33 studies between 1970 and 2000 found thirteen-fold lower rates of suicide and reported attempts during long-term lithium treatment than without it or after it was continued.

My personal interest in the study of lithium developed when I worked with the Medical Research Council, Metabolic Unit, at the Royal Edinburgh Hospital in 1978. Whilst I was impressed with its dramatic and almost curative effects in bipolar illness, I was also intrigued with its lack of efficacy in some patients. This observation prompted me to study predictors of response in an attempt to identify sub-groups of patients in relation to response to lithium including those who were lithium-resistant who could be spared exposure to it.

This review will focus on prediction of response to lithium in the acute treatment of mania, depression and to its prophylactic effects in recurrent affective disorders.

General considerations

Before reviewing the evidence for the effective use of various predictors of response to lithium it is important to address a number of issues. Firstly there is the issue of definition of response which ranges from complete success when no further episodes are observed to the other extreme of total lack of efficacy. Secondly there are qualitative and quantitative measures of response. In our studies, we have used the affective morbidity index (AMI) which is a composite index of the severity and duration of affective episodes. A recent analysis of the already published data[5] showed that predictors of response were the same whether a qualitative (response/non-response) or quantitative measure of outcome (AMI) was used. Thirdly there is non-compliance in relation to prediction of response. Aagaard and Vestergaard[1], distinguished between predictors of non-compliance with lithium and true predictors of response in lithium-adherent patients. Fourthly there is the issue of consistency of response or non-response between episodes of illness which has not been adequately studied. Jefferson[22] identified a number of other issues including the specificity of predictors to response to lithium versus other treatments such as anticonvulsants; for example, poor response to lithium in dysphoric mania, co-morbid substance abuse and personality disorder. The selection of patients and its impact on outcome with more recent studies showing less efficacy for lithium than earlier studies[20].

Predictors of antimanic response

In a recent review, Jefferson[22] identified a number of putative predictors of response to lithium in acute mania. Clinical characteristics of mania are poor predictors of response to lithium and the earlier finding that manic patients with paranoid destructive features respond poorly to lithium was not confirmed in later studies. Severity of mania including mania with psychotic features is also not a reliable predictor of poor response. The most important predictor of response, however, is the presence of depressive symptoms with mania – particularly if these symptoms qualify for the diagnosis of major depressive episode. It was noted that mixed affective states occur in 40% of manic episodes[18] with a good response that is half of that in pure mania. The recent placebo-controlled study of lithium, divaloproex in mania suggested that even a modest level of pre-treatment depression-related symptoms is a robust predictor of lithium non-response and is associated with better response to divaloproex[33]. The search for biological predictors of response has been disappointing. Sullivan et al.[30], reported that good response to lithium was associated with higher platelet monoamine oxidase activity than poor response. Swann et al.[32] reported that lithium non-responders had higher ratios of urinary MHPG excretion. Stoll et al.[29] found that patients with a high RBC choline levels had a poor response to lithium, a finding which may be related to the notion that patients with high RBC choline levels were more severely ill than those with lower levels. Goodwin and Jamison[18], in reviewing the evidence, identified predictors of poor antimanic response to lithium: mixed affective state, substance misuse and a history of rapid cycles which appear to predict a good antimanic response to carbamazepine.

Predictors of antidepressant response

Overall, bipolar depression responds better to lithium than unipolar depression. Goodwin and Jamison[18], in a review of placebo-controlled studies, found good response to lithium in 79% of bipolar patients and in 36% of unipolar patients. Studies of personality factors showed distinguishing characteristics of patients on the MMPI who respond well to lithium. Goodwin and Jamison[18] also reviewed the evidence for personality predictors of lithium response. They noted that lithium compliance was not adequately controlled for as well as the affective state at the time of personality testing, diagnostic criteria and measures of outcome. Biological variables have not been shown to have predictive value for lithium. Studies of lithium augmentation for refractory depression did not identify any predictors of response[23].

Predictors of prophylactic response

For both the patient and the clinician, prediction of response for prophylactic lithium is more important than prediction of its antimanic and antidepressants effects: it spares those who are poor responders to lithium a long-term trial of a potentially hazardous treatment and identifies optimal alternative treatment. Reviews of the evidence identified the following predictors: Goodwin and Jamison[18]; Abou-Saleh[4]; Jefferson[22].

Diagnosis and clinical features

Bipolar illness responds better to lithium than unipolar illness and 'pure' bipolar illness responds better than schizoaffective illness. Within bipolar illness, bipolar I responds better than bipolar II illness. This is probably related to the higher occurrence of personality disorder and substance misuse in bipolar II than bipolar I illness. Mania with psychotic symptoms responds better than mania without such symptoms, whilst mania with depressive symptoms responds less well than 'pure' mania. Bipolar illness starting with a manic episode responds better than if the first episode was depression.

Frequency and sequence of episodes

Among bipolar patients, those with frequent episodes (rapid cycling patients) show a greater incidence of prophylaxis failure than those with non-rapid cycling illness. Similarly, patients with a higher frequency of recent hospital admissions had a higher incidence of treatment failure on lithium.

Depressive episodes of patients with rapid cycling illness are more resistant to lithium than manic episodes. The occurrence of rapid cycling is strongly related to the use of antidepressants in the treatment of bipolar depression.

Episode sequence has an impact on prophylactic response. Kukopulos et al.[24] showed that patients with the classic mania–depression–normal interval had more favourable response than those with mania–depression–normal interval whilst those with a continuous circular course, particularly short cycles, had a poor response. These findings were confirmed by other investigators[19]. Maj and colleagues[26] reported similar findings in a prospective study in which the course of illness was evaluated independently of lithium efficacy.

Early and acute response

Early response (within 6–12 months) strongly predicts long-term response to lithium. Dunner and colleagues[17] studied clinical predictors of prophylaxis failure in non-rapid cycling bipolar patients. Although none of the clinical variables studied predicted outcome, they observed that patients who received lithium had a failure rate similar to those on placebo in the first six months of treatment. A quarter of their patients had early failure of treatment (within three months), and that tended to predict failure during their continued lithium treatment. Studies, by the author[5,6], of the long-term outcome of recurrent affective disorder with lithium treatment showed that the most powerful predictor was empirical: outcome over the first six months and first year predicted long-term outcome over 2–14 years.

The few open studies that evaluated the relationship of acute antimanic or antidepressant response to lithium and prophylactic response reported an association[31].

Co-morbidity

Patients with recurrent affective disorders and co-morbid medical and psychiatric disorders respond less well than those without co-morbidity. The common co-morbid psychiatric disorders are substance misuse, anxiety disorders and personality disorders.

Among the clinical features of affective states investigated, marked psychomotor retardation was found to be associated with better response[17]. There is inconsistent evidence for an association between the presence of family history of bipolar illness and favourable response to lithium[11]. A family history of non-bipolar affective disorder was not, however, associated with a more favourable response[17]. Studying a combined group of bipolar and unipolar patients, Svetska and Nahumeck[31] noted a family history of endogenous psychosis or suicide in first-degree relatives to be significantly associated with good prophylactic response. The most convincing evidence that genetic heterogeneity affects response to lithium was presented by Mendlewicz[27] in a study of twins. A high concordance rate was found in bipolar monozygotic and dizygotic twin pairs in which one twin experienced a good long-term response to lithium. Prophylactic response was better in concordant that in discordant twins.

In both bipolar and unipolar patients, those with greater disturbance in their personality characteristics, including neuroticism, introversion, low drive, and low self-confidence, responded less well than those with less or no personality disturbance[5].

Patients with substance misuse co-morbidity are at a particularly high risk of relapse or lithium failure which is probably mediated by the associated mixed affective states and/or poor compliance.

It has been claimed that responders show premorbid mood liability, whereas non-responders have premorbid traits of chronic anxiety and obsessiveness. Social support is strongly associated with good treatment outcome, as demonstrated in a study of 60 bipolar patients by O'Connell and co-workers[28]. Aagaard and Vestergaard[1], in their two-year prospective study, showed non-adherence to treatment was mainly predicted by substance abuse and many earlier admissions. Non-response in those who adhered to treatment was mainly predicted by female sex, younger age, and a previous chronic course. A third of the population of patients studied, however, had a chronic illness and half showed social deterioration prior to starting lithium. Life events in the 12 months prior to starting lithium had no influence on outcome on lithium. They also found that those who relapsed had no more life events prior to their relapse than at other times.

Biological predictors

Suboptimal thyroid function and hypothyroidism have been related to prophylaxis failure: thyroid hypofunction was shown to occur in patients who suffered recurrences, including those who developed rapid cycling bipolar disorder. Moreover, Coppen and Swade[15] showed that patients with high TSH levels without hypothyroidism suffered greater affective morbidity during prophylaxis.

A study of biological predictors of response[7] showed no association between the dexamethasone suppression test and response. Serotonin transport into the platelet, however, predicted response: patients who had an increase in V_{max} had lower long-term morbidity than those with decreased V_{max} (Abou-Saleh et al.[8]).

Platelet monoamine oxidase (MAO) activity in bipolar patients was not associated with response to prophylactic lithium[2]. Good response was, however, observed in those with increased calcium binding to red blood cells[3]. An increase in the red blood cell/plasma lithium ratio and a low frequency of HLA-A3 antigen were shown to predict good response over two years in a study of 100 bipolar and unipolar patients[26].

Conclusion

The search for predictors of outcome has not been particularly rewarding, and the use of lithium remains empirical: a trial of lithium is the most powerful predictor of outcome. Multivariate analysis of predictors of response showed that most of the variation in prophylactic response was accounted for by three factors: the diagnosis, the quality of the symptoms-free interval and the recent frequency of episodes[21]. In our own studies in a series of 116 bipolar and unipolar patients who received prophylactic lithium for a mean of 5.9 years, we identified three predictors of outcome: diagnosis, personality factors and early response over the first year[5]. Clinical and psychological variables examined may be general correlates or predictors of outcome rather than specific to lithium. However, lithium remains a highly specific treatment for bipolar disorder. Clinical, psychological, and biological correlates of non-bipolar affective disorder that predict good response to lithium are also correlates of bipolar disorder: mood-congruent psychotic features, retarded-endogenous profile, cyclothymic personality, positive family history of bipolar illness, periodicity, and normality between episodes of illness.

References

1. Aagaard J, Vestergaard P (1990). Predictors of outcome in prophylactic lithium treatment: a 2 year prospective study. *J Affect Disord.* 18:259–266.
2. Abou-Saleh MT (1983). Platelet MAO, personality and response to lithium prophylaxis. *J Affective Disorders* 5:55–65.
3. Abou-Saleh MT (1980). *Prediction of lithium response in manic depressive illness*. M. Phil. Thesis, University of Edinburgh.
4. Abou-Saleh MT (1993). Who responds to prophylactic lithium therapy? *Br J Psychiatry* Suppl (21): 20–6.
5. Abou-Saleh MT, Coppen AJ (1990). Predictors of long-term outcome of mood disorder on prophylactic lithium. *Lithium* 1:27–35.
6. Abou-Saleh MT, Coppen A (1986). Who responds to prophylactic lithium? *J Affective Disorders* 10: 115–125.

7. Abou-Saleh MT, Coppen A (1989). The efficacy of low-dose lithium: clinical, Psychological and Biological correlates. *J Psychiat* 23(2): 157–162.
8. Abou-Saleh MT, Swade C, Coppen AJ (1992). Increased Platelet 5-HT Transport is associated with Decreased Morbidity During Lithium Prophylaxis. *Lithium* 3, 301–304.
9. Baldessarini RJ, Tondo L, Hennen J (2001). Treating the suicidal patient with bipolar disorder. Reducing suicide risk with lithium. *Ann N Y Acad Sci* 932:24–38; discussion 39–43.
10. Burgess S, Geddes J, Hawton K, Townsend E, Jamison K, Goodwin G (2001). Lithium for maintenance treatment of mood disorders (Cochrane Review). *Cochrane Database Syst Rev.* 3;CD003013.
11. Carroll BJ (1979). Prediction of treatment outcome with lihtium. *Arch Gen Psychiatry* 36:870–878.
12. Coppen A (1994). Depression as a lethal disease: prevention strategies. *J Clin Psychiatry* 55: 37–45.
13. Coppen A, Abou-Saleh MT (1988). Lithium therapy: from clinical trials to practical management. *Acta Psychiatr. Scand* 78: 754–762.
14. Coppen A, Farmer R (1998). Suicide mortality in patients on lithium maintenance therapy. *J Affect Disord* 50(2–3)261–7.
15. Coppen A, Swade C (1986). *Reduced Lithium Dosage Improves Prophylaxis A Possible Mechanism. New Results in Depression Research* (Eds. H. Hippius et al.) Springer-Verlag Berlin Heidelberg 126–130.
16. Dickson WE, Kendell RE (1986). Does maintenance lithium therapy prevent recurrences of mania under ordinary clinical conditions? *Psychol. Med* 16(3): 521–30.
17. Dunner DL, Fleiss JL, Fieve RR (1976). Lithium carbonate prophylaxis failure. *Br J Psychiatry*, 129: 40–44.
18. Goodwin FK, Jamison KR (1990). *Manic-Depressive Illness*. New York, Oxford University Press.
19. Grof E, Haag M, Grof P, Haag H (1987). Lithium response and the sequence of episode polarities: preliminary report on a Hamilton sample. *Prog Neuropsychopharmacol Biol Psychiatry* 11(2–3): 199–203.
20. Grof P (1998). Has the effectiveness of lithium changed? Impact of the variety of lithium's effects. *Neuropsychopharmacology* 19(3):183–188.
21. Grof P, Alda M, Grof E, Fox D, Cameron P (1993). The Challenge of predicting response to stabilising lithium treatment. The importance of patient selection. *Br J Psychiatry Suppl.* Sept (21) 16–9.
22. Jefferson JW (1995). *Lithium in predictors of Treatment Response in Mood Disorders*. P J Goodnick (ed.) 95–117.
23. Johnson FN (1991). Lithium augmentation therapy for depression. *Reviews in Contemporary Pharmacotherapy* 2:1–52.
24. Kukopulos A, Reginaldi D, Laddomada P, Floris G, Serra G, Tondo L (1980). Course of the manic-depressive cycle and changes caused by treatment. *Pharmakopsychiatr Neuropsychopharmakol* 13(4):156–67.
25. Macritchie KA, Geddes JR, Scott J, Haslam DR, Goodwin GM. Valproic acid, valproate and divalproex in the maintenance treatment of bipolar disorder (Cochrane Review). *Cochrane Database Syst Rev.* 3:CD003196.
26. Maj M, Del Vecchio M, Starace F et al. (1984). Prediction of affective psychoses response to lithium prophylaxis: the role of socio-demographic, clinical, psychological and biological variables. *Acta Psychiatr Scand* 69:37–44.
27. Mendlewicz J (1979). Prediction of treatment outcome: family and twin studies in lithium prophylaxis and the question of lithium red blood cell/plasma ratios, in Lithium: Controversies and Unresolved Issues. (Eds by Cooper TB, Gershon S, Kline NS, Schou M). Amsterdam, *Exerpta Medica*. 226–240.
28. O'Connell RA, Mayo JA, Flatow L, Cuthbertson B, O'Brien BE (1991). Outcome of bipolar disorder on long-term treatment with lithium. *Br J Psychiatry* 159:123–9.
29. Stoll AL, Cohen BM, Snyder MB, Hanin I (1991). Erythrocyte choline concentration in bipolar disorder: a predictor of clinical course and medication response. *Biol Psychiatry* 15; 29(12): 1171–80.
30. Sullivan JL, Cavenar JO, Maltbie A et al., (1977). Platelet-monoamine-oxidase activity predicts response to lithium in manic-depressive illness. *Lancet* 2: 1325–1327.
31. Svetska J, Nahumeck K (1975). The result of lithium therapy in acute phases of affective psychoses and some other prognostical factors of lithium prophylaxis. *Act Nerv Super (Praha)* 17:270–271.
32. Swann AC, Koslow SH, Katz MM et al., (1987). Lithium carbonate treatment of mania: cerebrospinal fluid and urinary monoamine metabolites and treatment outcome. *Arch Gen Psychiatry* 44:345–354.

33. Swann AC, Bowden CL, Morris D, Calabrese JR, Petty F, Small J, Dilsaver SC, Davis JM, *et al.*, (1997). Depression during mania. Treatment response to lithium or divalproex. *Arch Gen Psychiatry* 54(1): 37–42.

Chapter 5
Focus on Chlorpromazine

Dr Samuel Vovnik and Dr Ben Green

Chlorpromazine is an aliphatic phenothiazine. It was developed at the laboratories Rhône-Poulenc/Specia in 1950. Credit for its development is shared between a number of individuals. The army surgeon Laborit, while looking for agents to prevent surgical shock, noted the calming and sedative properties of promethazine. He observed that patients given the drug prior to surgery, were relaxed and in relatively good spirits[15]. Its antihistaminic and sedative properties made it a suitable pre-surgical agent. It was decided at Rhône-Poulenc, to look for more antihistamines, in the same chemical class, but with a more pronounced central effect. In the Spring of 1951, the substance coded 4560RP was available. Using chlorpromazine, as 4560RP was later to be named, Laborit soon recognised its potential as a psychiatric agent. He noted its ability to calm patients and create a sense of detachment[2,3,15].

In early 1952, two psychiatrists, Delay and Deniker, administered chlorpromazine to acutely manic patients. They found the medication to be very effective and published a number of papers in rapid succession generating international interest for the new medication[6,7,8].

It was the efficacy with schizophrenic patients which was particularly impressive[16].

Its introduction heralded a revolution in the treatment of mental illness. It is the prototype for the many neuroleptic agents which were to follow.

Today, it remains an effective treatment particularly where sedation is required. However, with the advent of the second generation neuroleptics, mostly with more favourable side-effect profiles, many clinicians no longer consider it to be a drug of first choice in the treatment of psychosis.

Nevertheless, the Cochrane evidence-based review with 45 studies meeting its strict inclusion criteria concluded that chlorpromazine is effective in the treatment of schizophrenia, reduces relapse over six months to two years, and promotes a global improvement in a person's symptoms and functioning[34].

Mechanism of action

Chlorpromazine blocks postsynaptic dopamine receptors in the mesolimbic system and increases dopamine turnover by blocking D_2 somatodendritic auto-receptors. Depolarisation blockade of dopamine tracts leads to a decrease in dopamine neurotransmission[18,19].

It is the decrease in dopamine neurotransmission which has been correlated to the antipsychotic effect[20]. This is not an immediate process and peak antipsychotic effects may not occur for two to six months. This D_2 blockade is also responsible for the extrapyramidal and antiemetic effects of chlorpromazine.

The drug has strong alpha-adrenergic blocking activity which may cause postural hypotension, reflex tachycardia and occasionally a prolongation of the QT interval on the ECG. Anticholinergic activity is moderate and may manifest as occasional dry mouth, blurred vision, urinary retention and constipation[11].

Pharmacokinetics

Following oral administration, chlorpromazine is readily absorbed. However, bioavailability is variable due to first-pass metabolism by the liver. Food does not appear to affect oral bioavailability, which ranges from 19 to 51%. Some metabolism occurs in the gut wall but this is thought to be small. Very little renal excretion of the unchanged drug occurs[2,12,22].

There are many active and inactive metabolites. Effective plasma levels are decreased in the presence of delayed gastric emptying and by the use of drugs which decrease gastrointestinal motility. Chlorpromazine is highly bound to plasma albumin, approximately 90%[4]. It is widely distributed throughout the body, crossing the blood–brain barrier, the placenta and is distributed into milk. It is not dialysable. It can be administered intramuscularly and rectally. IM administration bypasses much of the first-pass effect and higher plasma concentrations are achieved. The onset of action is fastest for intramuscular administration (about 15 to 30 minutes). Onset of action for oral is 30 to 60 minutes and rectal, 45 to 90 minutes. The half-life is about 30 hours.

Indications

It can be used in the management of schizophrenia and other psychotic illnesses including the manic phase of manic depressive illness[17]. Its sedative nature can be used therapeutically in disturbed patients and as short-term adjunctive management of severe anxiety and psychomotor agitation[17].

It is also useful in the management of intractable hiccup, and in the treatment of nausea and vomiting due to stimulation of the chemoreceptor trigger zone.

It can be useful in a proportion of migraine attacks[32].

In a strange twist of fate that mirrors the chance finding that chlorpromazine is antipsychotic, recent research has suggested that it and other phenothiazines have antituberculous activity, and may come into their own with multi-drug resistant tuberculosis[31]. (This also echoes the strange cross-fertilisation of ideas between TB medicine and psychiatry with isoniazid/MAOIs, and the development of group therapy from TB patient support groups).

Contraindications

Chlorpromazine should not be given in comatose or depressed states due to its CNS depressant effect.

It should also be avoided in cases of blood dyscrasia, bone marrow depression liver damage and phaeochromocytoma. It should also be avoided in children or adolescents with signs or symptoms suggestive of Reye's Syndrome. The antiemetic effect can mask the signs while the CNS effect can be confused with the signs of Reye's syndrome.

Precautions

Chlorpromazine must be used with caution in patients who suffer with cardiovascular and cerebrovascular disease. An alpha-adrenergic blocking agent, it may cause an increased pulse rate and postural hypotension. The elderly are at particular risk[11].

Chlorpromazine has a direct negative inotropic action. It prolongs PR and QT intervals, blunts the T-wave and depresses the S–T segment. These changes are due to disturbances in repolarisation.

Use caution in patients who are spending time in hot climates. The sensitivity and adaptation to changes of environmental temperature may be impaired. Heat stroke and fatal hyperthermia are possible complications[11].

Chlorpromazine may lower the seizure threshold in patients with epilepsy. This effect becomes pronounced when other threshold-lowering drugs are combined with chlorpromazine.

Agranulocytosis occurs in some patients. Most reported cases occurred between the fourth and tenth week of treatment. If the patient negotiates three months without agranulocytosis, then it is unlikely to develop. Look out for the appearance of sore throat, fever and weakness. If these symptoms occur, discontinue the drug and perform a full white cell and differential counts.

Chlorpromazine-sensitive patients may have a cellular defect involving the final step of DNA synthesis, which limits incorporation of thymidine triphosphate into DNA. This reaction is associated with the production of bone marrow insufficiency in a patient who is believed to have a limited proliferative potential of bone marrow cells, which limit compensatory bone marrow response during treatment with a drug which ordinarily has limited bone marrow toxicity[10].

Chlorpromazine should be avoided in liver disease. In patients with hepatic precoma encephalopathy may be precipitated, due to altered brain sensitivity and respiratory depression[11].

If icterus or bilirubinemia occur discontinue the drug and perform liver function tests. A cholestatic hepatitis reaction occurs. This is not frequent and not related to dosage. Upon re-exposure about half of the sensitive individuals will have another reaction. Recovery is the rule once chlorpromazine is withdrawn.

For patients who are receiving the drug over a

prolonged period, regular ophthalmologic exams are recommended. Pigmentary retinopathy may occur particularly with high dosage over a prolonged period of time. Ocular changes appear to be positively correlated with severe photosensitivity responses to chlorpromazine.

Structure

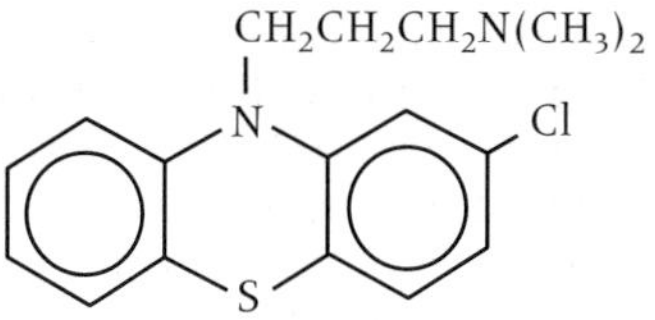

Figure 5.1: *Chlorpromazine is a tricyclic amine containing compound.*

Interactions

Interaction with other drugs is varied and ranges from minor side-effect enhancement to potentially serious complications. A number of commonly used drugs will affect the rate of metabolism of chlorpromazine requiring the dose prescribed to be adjusted[13].

Some of these are summarised in Table 5.1.

Side-effects

Chlorpromazine gives a wide range of side-effects. Many of these are minor and are seldom severe enough to call for a discontinuation of treatment. Recognised effects include drowsiness, blurred vision, dry mouth, pallor of the skin, skin rashes, tiredness and weakness, hypothermia and photosensitivity. The patient should be warned about dizziness and postural hypotension, as an unexpected dizzy spell may cause a fall. Generally, postural hypotension becomes less marked with continued treatment[11].

Extrapyramidal symptoms, including tardive dyskinesia on prolonged administration, can be problematic[25]. Akathisia is particularly unpleasant for the patient and is often a cause of poor compliance[9]. Starting at low doses and gradually increasing up to an effective dose lessens the risk of extrapyramidal side-effects[25].

Given intramuscularly, chlorpromazine may cause irritation at the injection site. The site of injection should be varied to avoid nodule formation.

Cholestatic jaundice is more common in women and usually resolves when the drug is discontinued. It is a rare side-effect. The drug must be stopped if it occurs.

Blood dyscrasias are a rare but serious complication, probably as a result of immunomodulation[29]. Immune-related side-effects may also include an SLE-like reaction. The mechanism for this may follow chlorpromazine mediated apoptosis in human lymphoblasts via intracellular signalling cascades[33].

The relative risk of developing cataracts on long-term chlorpromazine at daily doses of 300 mg or greater is 8.8[30].

Chlorpromazine has been retrospectively linked, along with other antipsychotics, to myocarditis or cardiomyopathy in a few patients[28].

Table 5.1: *Drug interactions of chlorpromazine.*

Drug	Interactions described
Ace inhibitor and other anti-hypertensives	Severe postural hypotension
Anticholinergic agents	Anticholinergic side-effects enhanced
CNS depressants	CNS depression enhanced
Beta-blockers	Risk of arrhythmia
Anti-arrhythmics	Paradoxically may increase risk of arrhythmia
Anaesthetic agents	Hypotensive effect enhanced
Tricyclic antidepressants	Increased risk of tardive dyskinesia
Antacids containing aluminium hydroxide and magnesium trisilicate	Reduce serum level
Lithium	Reduces serum levels
Tobacco	Reduces serum levels

Other side-effects reported include weight gain, and via prolactin – amenorrhea, galactorrhoea and impotence. In addition, chlorpromazine has an effect on functions of performance. Many patients report slower and confused thinking, difficulties in concentrating and feelings of clumsiness[11,14].

The recent Cochrane Review considers the large number of side effects choosing to highlight sedation (RR 2.4 CI 1.7-3.3, NNH 6 CI 4-8), acute movement disorders (RR 3.1 CI 1.3-7.6, NNH 24 CI 14-77), parkinsonism (RR 2.6 CI 1.2-5.4, NNH 10 CI 8-16) and fits (RR 2.4 CI 0.4-16) symptomatic hypotension (RR 1.9 CI 1. 3-2.6, NNH 12 CI 8-22) and significant weight gain (RR 4.4 CI 2.1-9, NNH 3 CI 2-5)[34].

Dosage

The average daily oral dose is 50 to 150 mg in 2–4 divided doses. Occasionally it is given in higher doses, up to 900 mg per day. It may take months for the optimum therapeutic effect to occur. Once symptoms are controlled the dosage should be gradually reduced to the lowest effective level for maintenance.

Caution should be exercised when using chlorpromazine in the elderly. They are more susceptible to CNS depression, hypotension and complications due to drug interactions.

Chlorpromazine may be administered parentally. The usual single dose varies between 25 to 50 mg. The risk of postural hypotension is increased with IM administration. This effect is enhanced with doses above 50 mg.

Although unlicensed in the UK, suppository preparations do exist and can be given in doses of 100 to 300 mg daily.

Conclusion

Even after 50 years, chlorpromazine continues to hold a place in the neuroleptic arsenal. It has the advantage of familiarity through time. Arguably, it has not been superseded in terms of efficacy, however side-effects, particularly the frequently occurring extrapyramidal ones, can impact greatly on the patient's quality of life. The newer atypical antipsychotics bring with them their own problems and have not yet driven the older typical ones out of clinical practice completely.

The impact of the discovery of chlorpromazine cannot be underestimated. Through its action on the dopamine pathway we have come some way in understanding the neurochemical processes involved in psychosis[20]. Socially its introduction was an important factor in the great fall of the asylum population in the latter half of the 20th century.

References

1. Carlton, PL, Marowotz P. Dopamine and Schizophrenia: an analysis of the theory. *Neuroscience and Biobehavioural Review*, 8:137, 1984.
2. Cooper SF, Abert JM, Hillel J, Caille G. Plasma-level studies of chlorpromazine following administration of chlorpromazine hydrochloride and chlorpromazine embonate in chronic schizophrenics. *Current Therapeutic Research*, 15:73, 1973.
3. Creese I, Burt D, Snyder SH. Biochemical actions of neuroleptic drugs: Focus on dopamine receptor. In, *Handbook of Psychopharmacology*, Vol. 10. (Iversen LL, Iversen SD, Snyder SH, eds.) Plenum Press, New York, 1978, pp. 37–89.
4. Dahl SG, Strandjord RE. Pharmacokinetics of chlorpromazine after single and chronic dosage. *Clinical Pharmacology and Therapeutics*, 21: 437, 1977.
5. Davis JM, Casper R. Antipsychotic drugs: Clinical pharmacology and therapeutic use. *Drugs*, 14: 260, 1977.
6. Delay J, Deniker P. Les neuropligiques en therapeutique psychiatrique. *Therapie*, 8:347–364, 1953.
7. Delay J, Deniker P. Trente-huit cas de psychoses traitees par la cure prolongee et continue de 4560 RP. Le Conqres des Al. et Neurol. De laque Fr. In, *Compte rendu du Conqres. Masson et Cie*, Paris, 1952.
8. Delay J, Deniker P, Harl JM. Utilisation en therapeutique psychiatrique d'une phenothiazine d'action centrale elective (4560RP). *Ann. Med-Psychol.*, 110:112–117, 1952.
9. Drake RE, Erlich H. Suicide attempts associated with akathisia. *American Journal of Psychiatry*, 142:499–501, 1985.
10. DuComb L, Baldessarini RJ. Timing and risk of bone marrow depression by psychotropic drugs. *Am. J. Psychiatry*, 134:1294–1295, 1977.
11. Edwards JG The untoward effects of antipsychotic drugs: Pathogenesis and management. In *The Psychopharmacology and Treatment of Schizophrenia* (eds. PB Bradley & SR Hirsch), pp. 403–441. Oxford: British Association for Psy-

chopharmacology Monograph, Oxford University Press, 1986.
12. Hollister LE, Curry SH, Derr JE, Kanter SL. Studies of delayed action medication V, Plasma levels and urinary excretion of four different dosage forms of chlorpromazine. *Clinical Pharmacology and Therapeutics*, 11:49, 1970.
13. Kaufman JS. Drug interactions involving psychotherapeutic agents. In, *Drug treatment of Mental Disorders*. (Simpson, L. L. ed). Raven Press, New York, 1976, pp. 289–309
14. King DJ. The effect of neuroleptics on cognitive and psychomotor function. *British Journal of Psychiatry*, 157:799–811, 1990.
15. Laborit H, Huquenard P, Alluime R. Un nowveau stabilisateur veqetatif (le 4560 R.P.). *Presse Med*, 60:206–208, 1952.
16. Labhardt F. Die Larqactil therapie bei Schizophrenien und anderen pscyhotischen Zustanden. *Schwreiz. Arch. Neurol. Psychiatr.*, 73:309–338, 1954.
17. Lehmann HE, Hanrahan GE. Chlorpromazine. New inhibiting agent for psychomotor excitement and manic states. *Archives of Neurology and Psychiatry*, 71:227–237, 1954.
18. Losonczy MF, Davidson M, Davis KL. The dopamine hypothesis of schizophrenia. In, *Psychopharmacology. The Third Generation of Progress*. (Melzer HY, ed.) Raven press, New York, 1987, pp. 715–726.
19. Mackay AVP, Iverson LL, Rossor M, *et al*. Increased brain dopamine and dopamine receptors in schizophrenia. *Archives of General Psychiatry*, 39:991–997, 1982.
20. Matthysse S. Antipsychotic drug actiersia, Federation Proceedings, 32, 200–205, 1973.
21. Meltzer HY, Goode DJ, Fanq VS. The effect of psychotropic drugs on endocrine function. In, *Psychopharmacology: A Generation of Progress*. (Lipton MA, DiMascio A, Killam KF, eds.) Raven Press, New York, 1978 pp. 509–529.
22. Rivera-Calimlin L, Naurallah H, Strauss J, Lasaqna L. Clinical response and plasma levels. Effect of dose, dosage schedules and drug interactions on plasma chlorpromazine levels. *American Journal of Psychiatry*, 133:646, 1976.
23. Spiegal, Rene: *Psychopharmacology an Introduction*, 3rd edition. John Wiley and Sons, 1996.
24. Tarsy D, Baldessarmi RJ, Clinical and pathophysiologic features of movement disorders induced by psychotherapeutic agents. In, *Movement Disorders*, (Shah, N., and Donald, A., eds.) Plenum Press, New York, 1986 pp. 365–389.
25. Swazey JP. *Chlorpromazine in Psychiatry: A study in therapeutic innovation*. M.I.T. Press, Cambridge, MA, 1974.
26. Coulter DM, Bate A, Meyboom RH, Lindquist M, Edwards IR. Antipsychotic drugs and heart muscle disorder in international pharmacovigilance: data mining study. *BMJ*, 322(7296): 1207–9, May 19, 2001.
27. Pollmacher T, Haack M, Schuld A, Kraus T, Hinze-Selch D. Effects of antipsychotic drugs on cytokine networks. [Review] [154 refs] *Journal of Psychiatric Research*, 34(6):369–82, 2000 Nov–Dec. 21104742.
28. Ruigomez A, Garcia Rodriguez LA, Dev VJ, Arellano F, Raniwala J. Are schizophrenia or antipsychotic drugs a risk factor for cataracts? *Epidemiology*, 11(6):620–3, 2000.
29. Bettencourt MV, Bosne-David S, Amaral L. Comparative in vitro activity of phenothiazines against multidrug-resistant Mycobacterium tuberculosis. *International Journal of Antimicrobial Agents*, 16(1):69–71, 2000.
30. Kelly AM. Migraine: pharmacotherapy in the emergency department. *Emergency Medicine Journal*, 17(4):241–5, 2000.
31. Hieronymus T, Grotsch P, Blank N, Grunke M, Capraru D, Geiler T, Winkler S, Kalden JR, Lorenz HM. Chlorpromazine induces apoptosis in activated human lymphoblasts: a mechanism supporting the induction of drug-induced lupus erythematosus?. *Arthritis & Rheumatism*, 43(9):1994–2004, 2000.
32. Thornley B, Adams CE, Awad G. Chlorpromazine versus placebo for schizophrenia. [Review] *Cochrane Database of Systematic Reviews* [computer file], (2):CD000284, 2000.

Chapter 6
Focus on Haloperidol

Professor Borwin Bandelow

Summary

Since its introduction 43 years ago the butyrophenone derivative haloperidol has been one of the most prescribed neuroleptics. It is being used in many psychiatric and neurological syndromes. Haloperidol has strong antipsychotic properties. It is associated with relatively strong extrapyramidal side-effects but has fewer sedating and autonomic side-effects than medium or low potency neuroleptics. In spite of the advantages of the atypical antipsychotics developed in the recent years which include lower liability for extrapyramidal effects and better efficacy in negative syndromes, the typical compound haloperidol will still play a major role in the treatment of schizophrenia.

Introduction

Haloperidol is probably the mostly investigated neuroleptic drug (13517 references in MEDLINE). It was developed by the Janssen-Cilag laboratories in Belgium and marketed in 1959. Oral, intravenous, intramuscular forms and a depot preparation (haloperidol decanoate) are available. Before the introduction of the atypical antipsychotics haloperidol was one of the most important drugs for the treatment of schizophrenia[5]. It is available in most countries.

Dosage regime

The dosage of haloperidol is highly variable and dependent of the patient's diagnosis, severity of illness and his individual reaction. Dosage of haloperidol cannot follow a certain schedule and must be titrated individually. While doses between 1.5 and 3 mg/day are sufficient for non-psychotic disorders, doses up to 100 mg/day are sometimes given in severe cases of schizophrenia and mania. Also, very high doses up to 300 mg have been used[62], but are not recommended for routine use. The highest dose a patient ever received was 1000 mg/day[22] which by no means is recommended but demonstrates the large therapeutic range of the drug.

The daily dose can be given in 1 to 3 dosages per day.

The following dosage regimen is recommended:

- For acute psychotic and catatonic syndromes, manic, schizophrenic and organic psychoses, mania and agitation states the dose should be started with 5–10 mg orally, IV or IM It can be titrated up to 60 mg parenterally or 100 mg orally for 24 hours. After remission of acute symptoms, 3–15 mg/day orally or more should be given. In delirious and organic syndromes a starting dose of 1–2 mg/day may already be sufficient.
- Agitated or hostile patients should be treated with 5–10 mg IM or IV. Injections may be repeated after 30 minutes.
- Dyskinetic syndromes and tics nerveux (such as Chorea Huntington, Gilles de la Tourette syndrome): start with 1 mg to a maximum dose of 40 mg/day orally.
- Children over 4 years: start with 0.025 mg/kg/day, maximum dose 0.2 mg/kg/day body weight.
- Nausea and vomiting: 1–3 mg orally, IV or IM.
- Non-psychotic syndromes: 0.5–2 mg orally.
- Dosage for children over 3 years: start with 0.025–0.5 mg/kg/day body weight, maximum dose 0.2 mg/kg/day body weight. For non-psychotic syndromes (such as hyperkinetic syndrome, autism) low dosages are recommended.
- For elderly patients, especially the ones with organic brain syndromes, very low dosages are recommended, starting with 0.5–1.5 mg/day. Elderly patients may have a higher liability for developing extrapyramidal syndromes and tardive dyskinesia.

Also, sedating effects and orthostatic hypotension may occur.
- The drug is available as a depot preparation (haloperidol decanoate) which is given in 4-week intervals. The starting dose is 12.5–50 mg/4 weeks. When changing from oral to depot medication, the fifteen-fold of the previous oral daily dose should be given for 4 weeks.

Structure*

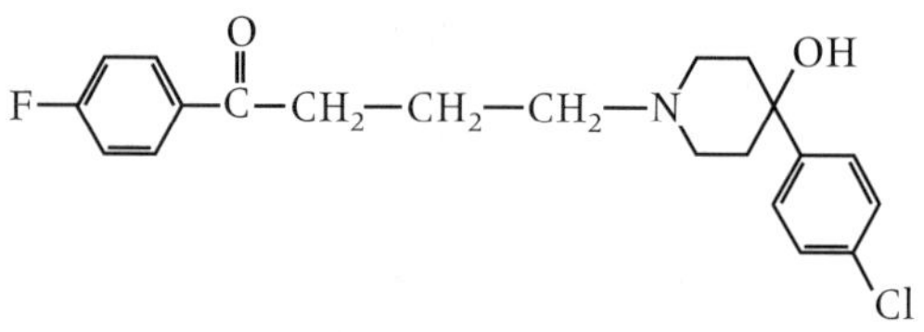

Figure 6.1: The haloperidol molecule.

Binding profiles

Haloperidol mainly blocks dopamine D_2 receptors. The affinity to serotonin receptors, α-adrenoceptors and sigma receptors is only moderate. Only in extremely high doses haloperidol can also have anticholinergic and antihistaminergic effects[48]. Prolactin increase may be substantial.

Clinical indications

Schizophrenia

Over 51 double-blind studies have shown the efficacy of haloperidol in schizophrenic psychoses (Table 6.1). In most of these studies haloperidol was at least equivalent to comparator drugs. Haloperidol is the reference drug for comparing new antipsychotic compounds with regard to positive schizophrenic symptoms. This explains why more studies have been conducted with haloperidol than with any other antipsychotic drug.

Organic psychoses

The antipsychotic effect of neuroleptics is unspecific. Not only schizophrenic patients, but also patients with organic psychoses can be treated with haloperidol[30,60,73]. Organic psychoses associated with dementia in the elderly may also be safely treated with haloperidol, as this drug causes less orthostatic, hypotensive and anticholinergic effects than other neuroleptics[24,77]. Haloperidol has also been used in the treatment of alcohol withdrawal. As all neuroleptics may lower seizure threshold, haloperidol should be combined with benzodiazepines in the treatment of patients with alcohol abuse.

Mania

Manic syndromes can also be treated with haloperidol[2,18,19,29,44,46,58,61]. Especially in cases in which very high doses are needed, haloperidol may be an alternative to other neuroleptics with pronounced autonomic side-effects.

Agitation states

Agitation states caused by psychotic and non-psychotic disorders can safely be treated with haloperidol[15,58,60]. Other medium or low potency drugs and some of the atypical compounds are less safe in treating severely agitated patients because they are associated with more orthostatic hypotension or cardiovascular or anticholinergic effects. Benzodiazepines are commonly used for sedating agitated patients. These drugs better tolerated by the patients but may carry the risk of respiratory depression.

Dyskinetic syndromes and tics nerveux

Dyskinetic syndromes, tics nerveux and Gilles de la Tourette syndrome are commonly treated with tiapride, pimozide or haloperidol[17,52]. As these syndromes often have an early onset in childhood, patients have to be exposed to the drug for many years, thus increasing the risk for developing tardive dyskinesia. New antipsychotics like ziprasidone may also be used in Tourette disorder[72], probably with a lower risk of developing tardive movement disorders.

Pharmacokinetics

The pharmacokinetics of haloperidol are shown in Table 6.2.

Adverse effects

Like many conventional high potency neuroleptics, haloperidol is associated with a high

---

* Haloperidol, 4' Fluor-4-[4-(4-chlorphenyl)-4-hydroxy-1-piperidyl]-butyrophenone, butyrophenone derivate

Chapter 6: Focus on Haloperidol

Table 6.1: *Haloperidol in schizophrenic psychoses (double-blind studies). > superior to; < less extrapyramidal symptoms (EPS).*

Reference	N pat.	Efficacy	EPS
[10]	36	haloperidol > placebo	haloperidol > placebo
[57]	69	haloperidol > placebo	haloperidol > placebo
[69]	12	haloperidol > placebo	haloperidol > placebo
[59]	27	haloperidol > placebo	haloperidol > placebo
[51]	388	risperidone = haloperidol > placebo	haloperidol > risperidone > placebo
[21]	41	haloperidol = amisulpride	haloperidol > amisulpride
[64]	39	haloperidol < amisulpride	haloperidol > amisulpride
[20]	40	haloperidol = amisulpride	haloperidol > amisulpride
[55]	191	haloperidol = amisulpride	haloperidol > amisulpride
[68]	319	haloperidol = amisulpride	haloperidol > amisulpride
[65]	40	haloperidol = bromperidol	haloperidol = bromperidol
[11]	47	haloperidol = bromperidol	haloperidol = bromperidol
[41]	164	haloperidol < bromperidol	haloperidol > bromperidol
[67]	58	haloperidol > chlorpromazine	haloperidol > chlorpromazine
[71]	50	haloperidol > chlorpromazine	haloperidol = chlorpromazine
[50]	30	haloperidol = chlorpromazine	haloperidol < chlorpromazine
[70]	50	haloperidol > chlorpromazine	haloperidol = chlorpromazine
[42]	91	haloperidol = clozapine	haloperidol > clozapine
[36]	40	haloperidol ≥ fluphenazine	haloperidol = fluphenazine
[61]	40	haloperidol = flupentixol	haloperidol = flupentixol
[53]	38	haloperidol = fluphenazine	haloperidol = fluphenazine
[45]	31	haloperidol = fluphenazine	haloperidol = fluphenazine
[7]	335	haloperidol = olanzapine > placebo	haloperidol > olanzapine > placebo
[78]	1996	haloperidol > olanzapine	haloperidol > olanzapine
[74]	32	haloperidol = perazine	haloperidol > perazine
[23]	29	haloperidol = perphenazine	haloperidol = perphenazine
[33]	20	haloperidol = pimozide	haloperidol > pimozide
[34]	30	haloperidol = pimozide	haloperidol < pimozide
[75]	22	haloperidol = pimozide	haloperidol = pimozide
[1]	361	haloperidol = quetiapine	haloperidol > quetiapine
[12]	62	haloperidol = risperidone	haloperidol > risperidone
[54]	35	haloperidol = risperidone	haloperidol > risperidone
[63]	1362	haloperidol = risperidone	haloperidol > risperidone
[81]	497	haloperidol = sertindole > placebo	haloperidol > sertindole = placebo
[35]	617	haloperidol = sertindole	haloperidol > sertindole
[28]	20 c.o.	haloperidol = sulpiride	haloperidol = sulpiride
[9]	32	haloperidol > tiospirone = thioridazine > placebo	?
[66]	40	haloperidol = thioridazine	haloperidol > thioridazine
[49]	21	haloperidol > thioridazine	haloperidol > thioridazine
[79]	86	haloperidol = thioridazine	haloperidol < thioridazine
[32]	21	haloperidol = trifluoperazine	haloperidol = trifluoperazine
[3]	40	haloperidol > trifluoperazine	haloperidol > trifluoperazine
[27]	45	trifluperidol > haloperidol = chlorpromazine	trifluperidol = haloperidol = chlorpromazine
[47]	26	haloperidol = zotepine	haloperidol > zotepine
[6]	30	haloperidol < zotepine	haloperidol > zotepine
[31]	90	ziprasidone = haloperidol	ziprasidone < haloperidol
[39]	301	ziprasidone = haloperidol	ziprasidone < haloperidol
[38]	63	haloperidol = zuclopenthixol	haloperidol = zuclopenthixol
[80]	64	haloperidol = zuclopenthixol	haloperidol = zuclopenthixol
[37]	49	haloperidol = zuclopenthixol	haloperidol = zuclopenthixol
[14]	40	haloperidol = zuclopenthixol	haloperidol = zuclopenthixol

Table 6.2: Pharmacokinetic parameters[8,13,25,26,40].

t_{max}	p.o. 3.2–6.0 hrs; IM 0.2–0.4 hrs
Bioavailability	tablets: 44–74% (mean: 60%); oral solution: 38–86% (mean: 58%)
Distribution half-life	p.o. 0.37–1.9 hrs; IV 0.19–0.23 hrs
Elimination half-life	p.o. 14.5–24.1 hrs; IV 14.1–26.2 hrs
Volume of distribution	9.5–21.7 l/kg
Clearance	33.0–49.2 l/kg
Serum protein binding	89–93%

liability for causing extrapyramidal symptoms (EPS). Many comparisons with atypical antipsychotics showed a higher frequency of EPS for haloperidol (Table 6.1). Thus, haloperidol should not be the first line treatment for the majority of patients. Only patients with severe psychoses who are non-responsive to atypical drugs, patients with co-morbid conditions or the ones who require depot medication should be treated with haloperidol.

Sedating effects may also occur frequently, although less than with many other neuroleptics.

Tardive dyskinesia may occur frequently after prolonged treatment. Occasionally, orthostatic hypotension and reflex tachycardia may occur at the start of treatment. Liver enzyme increases may occur. Occasionally, patients may complain about depressive syndromes[4]. Adverse effects due to prolactinaemia may occur, including galactorrhoea, amenorrhoea, gynaecomastia, weight gain and sexual dysfunctions. Rare adverse effects include blurred vision, hypersalivation, constipation, leucopenia, cholestatic hepatosis, neuroleptic malignant syndrome and others.

Interactions with other drugs

Like other neuroleptics, haloperidol is metabolised by the CYP1A2 system[56]. Haloperidol plasma levels may increase when the drug is combined with enzyme inhibitors such as fluvoxamine. CNS depression effects may be augmented when haloperidol is combined with other CNS-depressing drugs. Respiratory depression caused by polypeptide antibiotics may be increased by haloperidol. A combination with dopamine antagonists may increase extrapyramidal symptoms, combination with dopamine agonists may reduce the agonists' efficacy. The efficacy of some antihypertensive drugs may be increased. Combination with lithium may rarely lead to neurotoxic syndromes [16,76]. When combined with enzyme inducers such as carbamazepine, plasma concentration of haloperidol may be lowered[43]. Combination with adrenaline may lead to paradoxical hypotension.

Conclusion

Haloperidol is a pure D_2 blocking substance. This receptor binding profile is responsible for its excellent efficacy in severely ill psychotic patients. However, the drug is also associated with a high frequency of extrapyramidal symptoms. Because of its pure receptor binding profile, autonomic side-effects such as orthostatic hypotension, sedation, anticholinergic effects, cardiovascular effects and others are less frequent than with other neuroleptics.

Haloperidol may not be the drug of first choice for the average psychotic patients with medium severity of illness, good compliance and without comorbid conditions. In these patients atypical neuroleptics should be used. However, in very severe psychoses, aggressive and in hostile patients non-responsive to atypical drugs, in patients with cardiovascular problems, in the elderly and in patients with poor compliance haloperidol is still a valuable drug, as it is one of the safest of all neuroleptics.

References

1. Arvanitis LA, Miller BG. Quetiapine, an atypical antipsychotic: results from a multiple fixed dose, placebo-controlled study. Abstract, 149th Annual Meeting of the American Psychiatric Association, 1996.
2. Balant-Gorgia AE, Eisele R, Balant L, Garrone G. Plasma haloperidol levels and therapeutic

response in acute mania and schizophrenia. *Eur Arch Psychiatry Neurol Sci*, 1984;234:1–4.
3. Ban TA, Lehmann HE. Efficacy of haloperidol in drug refractory patients. *Int J Neuropsychiatry*, 1967;3:Suppl. 1:78–86.
4. Bandelow B, Müller P, Frick U, *et al*. Depressive syndromes in schizophrenic patients under neuroleptic therapy. ANI Study Group Berlin, Dusseldorf, Gottingen, Munich, Federal Republic of Germany. *Eur Arch Psychiatry Clin Neurosci*, 1992;241(5):291–5.
5. Bandelow B, Müller P, Rüther E. 30 Jahre Erfahrung mit Haloperidol. *Fortschr Neurol Psychiat*, 1991;8:297–321.
6. Barnas C, Stuppack CH, Miller C, Haring C, Sperner Unterweger B, Fleischhacker WW. Zotepine in the treatment of schizophrenic patients with prevailingly negative symptoms. A double-blind trial vs. haloperidol. *Int Clin Psychopharmacol*, 1992;7(1):23–7.
7. Beasley CM, Jr., Tollefson G, Tran P, Satterlee W, Sanger T, Hamilton S. Olanzapine versus placebo and haloperidol: acute phase results of the North American double-blind olanzapine trial. *Neuropsychopharmacology*, 1996;14(2):111–23.
8. Bianchetti G, Zarifan E, Poirier-Littre MF, Morsello PL, Deniker P. Influence of route of administration on haloperidol plasma levels in psychotic patients. *International Journal of Clinical Pharmacology, Therapy and Toxicology*, 1980;18:324–327.
9. Borison RL, Sinha D, Haverstock S, McLarnon MC, Diamond BI. Efficacy and safety of tiospirone vs. haloperidol and thioridazine in a double-blind, placebo-controlled trial. *Psychopharmacol Bull*, 1989;25(2):190–3.
10. Brandrup E, Kristjansen P. A controlled clinical test of a new psycholeptic drug (haloperidol). *J Ment Sci*, 1961;107:778–782.
11. Brannen JO, McEvoy JP, Wilson WH, *et al*. A double-blind comparison of bromperidol and haloperidol in newly admitted schizophrenic patients. *Pharmacopsychiatria*, 1981;14(4):139–40.
12. Ceskova E, Svestka J. Double-blind comparison of risperidone and haloperidol in schizophrenic and schizoaffective psychoses. *Pharmacopsychiatry*, 1993;26(4):121–4.
13. Cheng YF, Paalzow LK, Bondesson U, *et al*. Pharmacokinetics of haloperidol in psychotic patients. *Psychopharmacology Berl*, 1987;91(4):410–4.
14. Chouinard G, Safadi G, Beauclair L. A double-blind controlled study of intramuscular zuclopenthixol acetate and liquid oral haloperidol in the treatment of schizophrenic patients with acute exacerbation. *J Clin Psychopharmacol* 1994;14(6):377–84.
15. Clinton JE, Sterner S, Stelmachers Z, Ruiz E. Haloperidol for sedation of disruptive emergency patients. *Ann Emerg Med*, 1987;16(3):319–22.
16. Coffey CE, Ross DR. Treatment of lithium/neuroleptic neurotoxicity during lithium maintenance. *Am J Psychiatry*, 1980;137(6):736–7.
17. Connell PH, Corbett JA, Horne DJ, Mathews AM. Drug treatment of adolescent tiqueurs. A double-blind trial of diazepam and haloperidol. *Br J Psychiatry*, 1967;113(497):375–81.
18. Cookson JC, Moult PJ, Wiles D, Besser GM. The relationship between prolactin levels and clinical ratings in manic patients treated with oral and intravenous test doses of haloperidol. *Psychol Med*, 1983;13(2):279–85.
19. Cookson JC, Silverstone T, Williams S, Besser GM. Plasma cortisol levels in mania: associated clinical ratings and changes during treatment with haloperidol. *Br J Psychiatry*, 1985;146:498–502.
20. Costa e Silva JA. Etude comparative en double-insu amisulpride versus halopéridol dans le traitement des états psychotiques aigus. *Annales de Psychiatrie*, 1990;5:71–78.
21. Delcker A, Schoon ML, Oczkowski B, Gaertner HJ. Amisulpride versus haloperidol in treatment of schizophrenic patients – results of a double-blind study. *Pharmacopsychiatry*, 1990;23(3):125–30.
22. Denber HCB, Collard J. Differences de bioréactivité au Halopéridol entre deux groupes de psychotiques, américain et européen. *Acta Neurol Psychiat Belg*, 1962;62:577–588.
23. Dencker SJ, Gios I, Martensson E, *et al*. A long-term cross-over pharmacokinetic study comparing perphenazine decanoate and haloperidol decanoate in schizophrenic patients. *Psychopharmacology Berl*, 1994;114(1):24–30.
24. Devanand DP, Sackeim HA, Brown RP, Mayeux R. A pilot study of haloperidol treatment of psychosis and behavioral disturbance in Alzheimer's disease. *Arch Neurol* 1989;46(8):854–7.
25. Forsman A, Öhman R. Pharmacokinetic studies on haloperidol in man. *Curr Ther Res Clin Exp*, 1976;20(3):319–36.
26. Forsman A, Öhman R. Studies on serum protein binding of haloperidol. *Curr Ther Res Clin Exp*, 1977;21(2):245–55.
27. Fox W, Gobble F, Clos M. A clinical comparison of trifluperidol, haloperidol, and chlorpromazine. *Curr Ther Res*, 1964;4:409–15.

28. Gerlach J, Behnke K, Heltberg J, Munk Anderson E, Nielsen H. Sulpiride and haloperidol in schizophrenia: a double-blind cross-over study of therapeutic effect, side effects and plasma concentrations. *Br J Psychiatry*, 1985;147:283–8.
29. Gerle B. Haloperidol clinical experience. *Clin Trial J*, 1966;3:360–384.
30. Giannini AJ, Eighan MS, Loiselle RH, Giannini MC. Comparison of haloperidol and chlorpromazine in the treatment of phencyclidine psychosis. *J Clin Pharmacol*, 1984;24(4):202–4.
31. Goff DC, Posever T, Herz L, et al. An exploratory haloperidol-controlled dose-finding study of ziprasidone in hospitalized patients with schizophrenia or schizoaffective disorder. *Journal of Clinical Psychopharmacology*, 1998;18(4): 296–304.
32. Goldstein BJ, Clyde DJ. Haloperidol in controlling the symptoms of acute psychoses. II. A double-blind evaluation of haloperidol and trifluoperazine. *Curr Ther Res Clin Exp*, 1966;8(5): 236–40.
33. Gowardman M, Barrer B, Brown RA. Pimozide (R6238) in chronic schizophrenia: double blind trial. *New Zealand Med J*, 1973;Dec 12:487–91.
34. Haas S, Beckmann H. Pimozide versus Haloperidol in acute schizophrenia. A double blind controlled study. *Pharmacopsychiatria*, 1982;15(2): 70–4.
35. Hale A, van der Burght M, Wehnert A, Friberg HH. A European dose-range study comparing the efficacy, tolerability and safety of four doses of sertindole and one dose of haloperidol in schizophrenic patients. Poster, CINP Congress, Mebourne, Australia 1996.
36. Hall WB, Vestre ND, Schiele BC, Zimmermann R. A controlled comparison of haloperidol and fluphenazine in chronic treatment-resistant schizophrenics. *Dis Nerv Syst*, 1968;29(6):405–8.
37. Heikkila L, Eliander H, Vartiainen H, Turunen M, Pedersen V. Zuclopenthixol and haloperidol in patients with acute psychotic states. A double-blind, multi-centre study. *Curr Med Res Opin*, 1992;12(9):594–603.
38. Heikkila L, Laitinen J, Vartiainen H. Cis(Z)-clopenthixol and haloperidol in chronic schizophrenic patients – a double-blind clinical multi-centre investigation. *Acta Psychiatr Scand*, Suppl. 1981;294:30–8.
39. Hirsch S, Power A, Kissling W. A 28-week comparison of flexible-dose ziprasidone with haloperidol in outpatients with stable schizophrenia. *Congress of the American Psychiatric Association* (APA), Toronto, 1999.
40. Holley FO, Magliozzi JR, Stanski DR, Lombrozo L, Hollister LE. Haloperidol kinetics after oral and intravenous doses. *Clin Pharmacol Ther*, 1983;33(4):477–84.
41. Itoh H. A comparison of the clinical effects of bromperidol, a new butyrophenone derivative, and haloperidol on schizophrenia using a double-blind technique. *Psychopharmacol Bull*, 1985; 21(1):120–2.
42. Itoh H, Miura S, Yagi G, Sakurai S, Ohtsuka N. Some methodological considerations for the clinical evaluation of neuroleptics – comparative effects of clozapine and haloperidol on schizophrenics. *Folia Psychiatr Neurol Jpn* 1977; 31(1):17–24.
43. Jann MW, Ereshefsky L, Saklad SR, et al. Effects of carbamazepine on plasma haloperidol levels. *J Clin Psychopharmacol*, 1985;5(2):106–9.
44. Kelwala S, Ban TA, Berney SA, Wilson WH. Rapid tranquilization: a comparative study of thiothixene and haloperidol. *Prog Neuropsychopharmacol Biol Psychiatr*, 1984;8:77–83.
45. Kissling W, Möller HJ, Walter K, Wittmann B, Krueger R, Trenk D. Double-blind comparison of haloperidol decanoate and fluphenazine decanoate effectiveness, side-effects, dosage and serum levels during a six months' treatment for relapse prevention. *Pharmacopsychiatry*, 1985;18(3):240–5.
46. Klein E, Bental E, Lerer B, Belmaker RH. Carbamazepine and haloperidol v placebo and haloperidol in excited psychoses. A controlled study. *Arch Gen Psychiatry*, 1984;41(2):165–70.
47. Klieser E, Lehmann E, Tegeler J. Doppelblindvergleich von 3×75 mg Zotepin und 3×4 mg Haloperidol bei akut schizophrenen Patienten. *Fortschr Neurol Psychiatr*, 1991;59 Suppl. 1:14–7.
48. Leysen JE, Janssen PM, Schotte A, Luyten WH, Megens AA. Interaction of antipsychotic drugs with neurotransmitter receptor sites in vitro and in vivo in relation to pharmacological and clinical effects: role of $5HT_2$ receptors. *Psychopharmacology Berl*, 1993;112(1 Suppl):S40–54.
49. Luckey WT, Schiele BC. A comparison of haloperidol and trifluoperazine (a double-blind, controlled study on chronic schizophrenic outpatients). *Dis Nerv Syst*, 1967;28(3):181–6.
50. Man PL, Chen CH. Rapid tranquilization of acutely psychotic patients with intramuscular haloperidol and chlorpromazine. *Psychosomatics*, 1973;14(1):59–63.
51. Marder SR, Meibach RC. Risperidone in the treatment of schizophrenia. *Am J Psychiatry*, 1994;151(6):825–35.

52. McDougle CJ, Goodman WK, Leckman JF, Lee NC, Heninger GR, Price LH. Haloperidol addition in fluvoxamine-refractory obsessive-compulsive disorder. A double-blind, placebo-controlled study in patients with and without tics. *Arch Gen Psychiatry*, 1994;51(4):302–8.
53. McKane JP, Robinson AD, Wiles DH, McCreadie RG, Stirling GS. Haloperidol decanoate v. fluphenazine decanoate as maintenance therapy in chronic schizophrenic in-patients. *Br J Psychiatry*, 1987;151:333–6.
54. Min SK, Rhee CS, Kim CE, Kang DY. Risperidone versus haloperidol in the treatment of chronic schizophrenic patients: a parallel group double-blind comparative trial. *Yonsei Med J*, 1993;34(2):179–90.
55. Möller HJ, Boyer P, Fleurot O, Rein W. Improvement of acute exacerbations of schizophrenia with amisulpride: a comparison with haloperidol. PROD-ASLP Study Group. *Psychopharmacology Berl*, 1997;132(4):396–401.
56. Nemeroff CB, DeVane CL, Pollock BG. Newer antidepressants and the cytochrome P450 system. *Am J Psychiatry*, 1996;153(3):311–20.
57. Okasha A, Tewfik GI. Haloperidol: a controlled clinical trial in chronic disturbed psychotic patients. *Br J Psychiat*, 1964;110:56–60.
58. Oldham AJ, Bott M. The management of excitement in a general hospital psychiatric ward by high dosage haloperidol. *Acta-Psychiatr-Scand*, 1971;47(4):369–76.
59. Ota KY, Kurland AA. A double-blind comparison of haloperidol oral concentrate, haloperidol solutabs and placebo in the treatment of chronic schizophrenia. *J Clin Pharmacol New Drugs*, 1973;13(2):99–110.
60. Pakalnis A, Drake ME, Jr., John K, Kellum JB. Forced normalization. Acute psychosis after seizure control in seven patients. *Arch Neurol*, 1987;44(3):289–92.
61. Parent M, Toussaint C. Flupenthixol versus haloperidol in acute psychosis. *Pharmatherapeutica*, 1983;3(5):354–64.
62. Petit P, Blayac JP, Castelnau D, Billet J, Puech R, Pouget R. Utilisation de très fortes posologies d'halopéridol dans le traitement des épisodes psychotiques aigus. *L'encéphale*, 1987;13(3):127–0.
63. Peuskens J. Risperidone in the treatment of patients with chronic schizophrenia: a multinational, multi-centre, double-blind, parallel-group study versus haloperidol. Risperidone Study Group. *Br J Psychiatry*, 1995;166(6):712–26.
64. Pichot P, Boyer P. Etude multicentrique contrôlée en double insu: amisulpride (SolianR 200) versus halopéridol à forte dose dans les états psychotiques aigus. *Annales de Psychiatrie*, 1988;3:326–332.
65. Pöldinger W. Clinical experiences in an open and a double-blind trial. *Acta Psychiatr Belg*, 1978;78(1):96–101.
66. Prasad L, Townley MC. Haloperidol and thioridazine in treatment of chronic schizophrenics. *Dis Nerv Syst*, 1966;27(11):722–6.
67. Pratt JP, Bishop MP, Gallant DM. Trifluoperidol and haloperidol in treatment of acute schizophrenia. *Am J Psychiatry*, 1964;121:592–594.
68. Puech A, Fleurot O, Rein W, Amisulpride Study Group. Amisulpride, an atypical antipsychotic, in the treatment of acute episodes of schizophrenia: a dose-ranging study vs. haloperidol. *Acta Psychiat Scand*, 1998;98:65–72.
69. Rees L, Davis B. A study of the value of haloperidol in the management and treatment of schizophrenic and manic patients. *Int J Neuropsychiat*, 1965;1:263–5.
70. Reschke RW. Parenteral haloperidol for rapid control of severe, disruptive symptoms of acute schizophrenia. 1974;35:112–115.
71. Ritter RM, Davidson DE, Robinson TA. Comparison of injectable haloperidol and chlorpromazine. *Am J Psychiatry*, 1972;129(1):78–81.
72. Sallee FR, Kurlan R, Goetz CG, et al. Ziprasidone treatment of children and adolescents with Tourette's syndrome: a pilot study. *J Am Acad Child Adolesc Psychiatry*, 2000;39(3):292–9.
73. Sato M, Chen CC, Akiyama K, Otsuki S. Acute exacerbation of paranoid psychotic state after long-term abstinence in patients with previous methamphetamine psychosis. *Biol Psychiatry*, 1983;18(4):429–40.
74. Schmidt LG, Schüssler G, Kappes CV, Müller-Oerlinghausen B. Vergleich einer hoher dosierten Haloperidol-Therapie mit einer Perazin-Standard-Therapie bei akut schizophrenen Patienten. *Nervenarzt*, 1982;53(9):530–6.
75. Silverstone T, Cookson J, Ball R, et al. The relationship of dopamine receptor blockade to clinical response in schizophrenic patients treated with pimozide or haloperidol. *J Psychiatr Res*, 1984;18(3):255–68.
76. Spring G, Frankel M. New data on lithium and haloperidol incompatibility. *Am J Psychiatry*, 1981;138(6):818–21.
77. Tobin JM, Brousseau ER, Lorenz AA. Clinical evaluation of haloperidol in geriatric patients. *Geriatrics*, 1970;25(6):119–22.

78. Tollefson GD, Beasley CM, Jr., Tran PV, et al. Olanzapine versus haloperidol in the treatment of schizophrenia and schizoaffective and schizophreniform disorders: results of an international collaborative trial. *Am J Psychiatry* 1997; 154(4):457–65.
79. Weston MJ, Bentley R, Unwin A, Morris M, Harper MA. A comparative trial of haloperidol and thioridazine: management of chronic schizophrenia. *Aust N Z J Psychiatry*, 1973;7(1): 52–7.
80. Wistedt B, Koskinen T, Thelander S, Nerdrum T, Pedersen V, Molbjerg C. Zuclopenthixol decanoate and haloperidol decanoate in chronic schizophrenia: a double-blind multicentre study. *Acta Psychiatr Scand*, 1991;84(1):14–21.
81. Zimbroff DL, Kane JM, Tamminga CA, et al. Controlled, dose-response study of sertindole and haloperidol in the treatment of schizophrenia. Sertindole Study Group. *Am J Psychiatry*, 1997;154(6):782–91.

Chapter 7
Focus on Clozapine

Dr Miriam Naheed and Dr Ben Green

Summary

Clozapine is a dibenzodiazepine derivative and a truly atypical antipsychotic. Its therapeutic effects are probably mediated by dopaminergic and serotonergic activity. Although it appears to be the most effective antipsychotic drug for treatment-resistant schizophrenia, its general use is limited because of the risk of agranulocytosis.

Introduction

Clozapine is manufactured by Novartis pharmaceuticals and marketed under the trade name of Clozaril. Its structural formula is given in Figure 7.1.

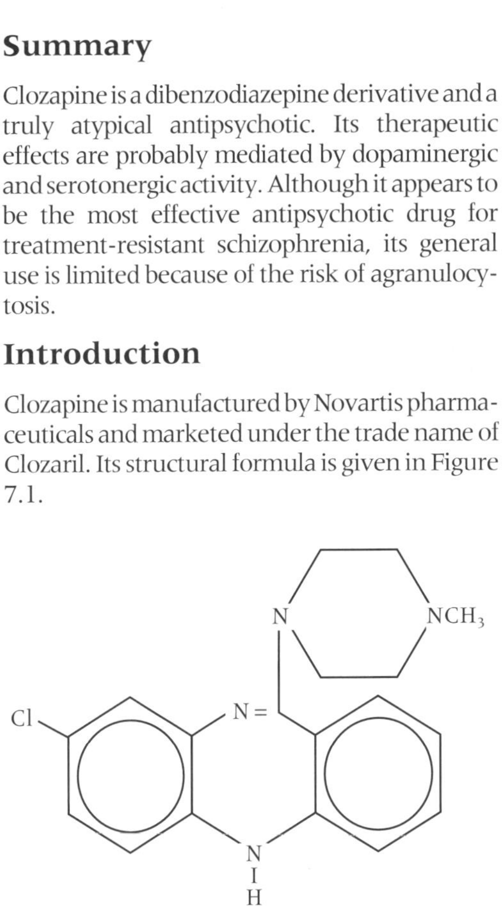

Figure 7.1: The structure of clozapine.

It is an atypical antipsychotic agent whose mode of action is thought to pertain to its interaction with dopaminergic and serotonergic neurotransmitter systems. Its clinical efficacy may depend on plasma clozapine concentrations, but its response rate varies widely. The response rate is anywhere between 30% and 100% of patients on short-term therapy, whereas, during long-term treatment, 60% of patients unresponsive to, or intolerant of, previous antipsychotics respond to clozapine. Significant improvements in both positive and negative psychotic symptoms, quality of life, social functioning and suicidality have been demonstrated.

It represents the first major advance in the treatment of schizophrenia since the advent of antipsychotics in the 1950s.

Although clozapine has been found to be the most effective antipsychotic drug for treatment-resistant schizophrenia, its use has been greatly limited because of the risk of agranulocytosis, which has, in fact, been shown to have a frequency which is less than 1%[1]. In balancing benefits against risks, it is worth noting that the suicide mortality rate in patients with schizophrenia not treated with clozapine is much higher than the mortality from agranulocytosis in the patients treated with clozapine[2,3]. With periodic blood monitoring, the agranulocytosis risk is 0.38%[1].

Background history

Clozapine was introduced in Europe in 1975. As a result of reports from Finland, where 16 patients out of 2260 exposed (0.7%) developed agranulocytosis and 8 (50%) of them subsequently died from secondary infections, the drug was voluntarily withdrawn from use. Following pressure from psychiatrists to reintroduce clozapine, trials in patients with treatment-resistant schizophrenia, under close haematological monitoring, were devised, which showed significant improvement in 30% of patients after six months[4,5]. Subsequent studies showed improvement in 61% of patients if treatment was continued for up to one year[6,7]. These data, together with a proposal for a national coordinated mandatory haematological monitoring service for all patients, enabled clozapine to be given a product licence in the UK in January 1990, and in Ireland in August 1993.

All patients treated with clozapine in the UK must register with the Clozaril Patient Monitoring Services (CPMS), so as to ensure that no patient can receive the drug without a recent satisfactory haematological result. It also helps guarantee that clozapine is stopped immediately if a patient develops a fall in the white cell count. Since the introduction of the CPMS, the incidence of agranulocytosis-related mortality has reduced tremendously.

Recent evidence based on a patient population of 6000 in the UK suggests that the risk of agranulocytosis decreases ten-fold from 0.73% during the first year of therapy to 0.07% after this[8].

Despite its proven benefits, clozapine is probably underprescribed because of its limited indication of treatment-resistant and treatment-intolerant schizophrenia and the negative perception relating to the risk of agranulocytosis.

Indications

Under the terms of its UK licence, clozapine should only be used for patients with schizophrenia who are unresponsive to two or more antipsychotics or who are intolerant of their neurological side-effects. Only psychiatrists registered with the manufacturer's Clozaril Patient Monitoring Services (CPMS) can prescribe it. Clozapine's beneficial use in several unlicensed disorders is being investigated, including psychosis secondary to dopaminergic therapy or coexisting psychiatric disorders in Parkinson's disease, other psychotic disorders, affective disorders, dyskinesias and related disorders, dementia, mental retardation, and polydipsia/hyponatraemia. There are a number of reports showing clozapine's dramatically beneficial effect in patients with severe personality disorder where all other treatment options have failed. These case reports and small studies show marked reduction in self-harming behaviour, aggression and intensive affective response in this patient group[9–12].

There is evidence to suggest that, used in schizophrenia, clozapine improves social functioning, occupational functioning and quality of life and that it may also reduce affective symptoms, hospitalisation, secondary negative symptoms and tardive dyskinesia.

Pharmacology

Clozapine is a prototype 'broad-spectrum' antagonist. Its binding profile is quite different from other antipsychotics both within and outside the dopaminergic system. It has relatively low affinity for D_2 receptors in the striatum, while its *in vitro* affinity for the D_4 receptors is approximately ten times greater than that for D_2 receptors, and it has also been shown to bind to the D_1, D_3 and D_5 receptors. Since D_4 density is highest in the frontal cortex and amygdala but relatively low in the basal ganglia, this may be the explanation for the efficacy of clozapine in alleviating the symptoms of schizophrenia without causing extrapyramidal side-effects. Clozapine has been recognised to show significant activity at a broad range of receptors outside the DA system. Of particular interest is its high affinity for 5-HT receptors, including $5-HT_2$, $5-HT_3$, $5-HT_6$ and $5-HT_7$ subtypes. Clozapine has high affinities for muscarinic A_1 and A_2 receptors, while it also has significant effects on GABA-ergic and glutamatergic mechanisms.

Pharmacokinetics and metabolism

After oral administration the drug is rapidly absorbed. There is extensive first-pass metabolism and only 27–50% of the dose reaches the systemic circulation unchanged.

Its plasma concentration has been observed to vary from patient to patient. Various individual factors may vary response such as smoking, hepatic metabolism, gastric absorption, age and, possibly, gender. Clozapine is rapidly distributed. It crosses the blood–brain barrier and is distributed in breast milk. It is 95% bound to plasma proteins. Steady-state plasma concentration is reached after 7–10 days. The onset of the antipsychotic effect can take several weeks, but maximum effect may require several months. In treatment-resistant schizophrenia, patients have been reported to continue to improve for at least two years after the start of clozapine treatment. Clozapine metabolises into various metabolites, out of which only norclozapine (a desmethyl metabolite) is pharmacologically active. The other metabolites do not appear to have clinically significant activity. Its plasma concentration declines in the biphasic manner, typical of oral antipsychotics, and its mean elimination half-life ranges from 6 to 33 hours. About 50% of a dose is excreted in urine and 30% in the faeces.

Dose

Clozapine is started from a dose of 12.5 mg/day. On day two the dose can be increased to 12.5 mg twice daily. If the patient is tolerating the clozapine, the dose can then be increased by 25 mg to 50 mg a day, until a dose of 300 mg a day is reached. This can usually be achieved in two to three weeks. Further dosage increases should be made slowly in increments of 50–100 mg each week. A dose of 450 mg/day or a plasma level of 350 mcg/l should be aimed for. The total clozapine dose should be divided and, if sedation is a problem, a larger proportion of the dose can be given at night[13].

Therapeutic efficacy

The efficacy of clozapine has been examined in a large number of studies since it was first introduced. There is a substantive number of randomised double-blind trials, in which clinical efficacy of clozapine in acutely psychotic and treatment-resistant schizophrenics has been rigorously examined.

Effect on positive and negative symptoms of schizophrenia

Both positive and negative symptoms of schizophrenia appeared to be improved with clozapine treatment. Negative symptoms improved in direct relation to positive symptoms in 40 schizophrenic patients after clozapine therapy for eight weeks[14]. Lieberman et al.[15] reported that negative symptoms responded to treatment approximately seven weeks after a decrease in positive symptoms in 84 patients with treatment-resistant schizophrenia. The results of these studies imply that the greater improvement in negative symptoms seen in patients receiving clozapine compared with those receiving classical antipsychotic agents may be associated with the greater improvement in positive symptoms and fewer extrapyramidal symptoms (which can mimic negative symptoms) in these patients, rather than an independent action on negative symptoms[16]. However, in a cohort of 36 patients with schizophrenia unresponsive to previous therapy, statistically significant reductions in Brief Psychiatric Rating Scale (BPRS) on withdrawal/retardation score were seen after six months' therapy with clozapine and psychosocial treatment in patients with high-negative/low-positive, as well as in those with high-negative/high-positive, symptoms[17].

Acute psychosis

Most of the studies found clozapine to be more effective than conventional neuroleptics in treating both positive, as well as negative, symptoms in acutely ill schizophrenics[18–20].

Treatment-resistant schizophrenia

Clozapine is still the only drug of proven efficacy in treatment-resistant schizophrenia[21,22]. The significant response of neuroleptic-resistant schizophrenia patients to clozapine validates its efficacy in this group[23]. Kane et al.[5], in their famous multicentre double-blind trial, compared chlorpromazine with clozapine in equivalent doses and found that 4% chlorpromazine vs. the 30% clozapine group responded by marked reduction in BPRS score (both positive and negative symptoms) in six weeks.

Lieberman et al.[15] reported that the response rate of clozapine was 50% among previously treatment-refractory patients and 76% among treatment-intolerant patients.

Objective measures have indicated a marked improvement in psychopathology, including negative symptoms such as blunted affect, emotional withdrawal and apathy[24,25]. Besides improvement of positive and negative symptoms, clozapine may improve organisation of thought, improve certain aspects of cognitive function and enable patients to resume functioning in a low normal range. In line with an improvement in overall psychopathology, treatment with clozapine is associated with improved compliance with medication regimen and less need for hospitalisation[26–28].

Effect of clozapine on aggressive behaviour

The improvement in aggressive behaviour among schizophrenic patients receiving clozapine has been an interesting finding in the clinical trials[29–35].

The question arises as to whether clozapine's efficacy derives from a specific anti-aggressive effect, or the reduction in violent behaviour merely reflects an overall improvement in psychosis. Buckley et al.[34] have addressed this issue by comparing the symptomatic response to clozapine in 30 institutionalised schizophrenic patients, 11 of whom displayed persistent violent behaviour before initial use of clozapine. Although the violent patients showed a dramatic reduction in aggression during six months of clozapine treatment, their overall response to measures on BPRS was comparable to that of non-violent patients. This suggests that the violent behaviour was not tightly coupled to the severity of illness *per se* and raises the possibility of a distinct anti-aggressive effect. Volavka et al.[31] in New York have also demonstrated the selective effect of clozapine on hostility that is above and beyond the improvement of psychosis. At present it is uncertain how clozapine could be incorporated in the pharmacological treatment of aggression. Its side-effects limit its broad use for patients with varying conditions and severity who also exhibit violent behaviour. However, in situations where violence is a severe problem, the benefit could outweigh the potential risk.

Drug and alcohol abuse

Clozapine significantly decreases the co-morbid use of alcohol and drugs in patients with schizophrenia, possibly by a reduction in the craving[36].

In one case study, a decrease in cocaine use after clozapine therapy was reported in a treatment-resistant 37-year-old male with schizoaffective disorder[37]. There are other reports of dramatic cessation of substance abuse, attenuated craving and improved psychosocial functioning during clozapine therapy[38]. Patients report a reduction in craving, which has been considered to be due to the differential effect of clozapine on dopamine neurotransmission in the nucleus accumbens, a region known to be involved in the neurobiology of craving.

Prevention of Suicide

Evidence is accumulating that clozapine is efficacious in reducing suicidality in schizophrenia. Meltzer, in the Clozapine and InterSept study[39], reported an 80–85% reduction in the incidence of suicide in neuroleptic-resistant patients prescribed clozapine. Walker et al.[40] reported the results of a retrospective analysis of mortality of 67,072 schizophrenic patients receiving clozapine in the interval between April 1st, 1991 and December 31st, 1993. The data were acquired from the clozaril national registry. Patients were classified as current, recent or past clozapine users. The striking finding was that of a dramatic reduction in the incidence of suicide among current users of clozapine. While the incidence of suicide in this cohort was 19% of overall mortality, the patients who committed suicide were primarily those who had stopped using clozapine.

Mood disorders

Clozapine has been shown to be effective in severe mood disorders. In a one-year randomised trial of clozapine versus treatment-as-usual among 39 bipolar patients, clozapine's superiority was evident within the first 6 months of treatment and was maintained throughout the duration of this study[41]. Zarate et al.[42] reported that, for schizoaffective disorder, 70% of patients achieved demonstrable improvement in symptoms with clozapine therapy. Clozapine has also been reported to be of benefit in psychotic depression[43].

Drug-induced psychosis in Parkinson's disease

A randomised, double-blind, placebo-controlled trial of low doses of clozapine (25–50 mg per day) in 60 patients over a period of 14 months showed significant improvement in drug-induced psychosis in Parkinson's disease, without worsening Parkinsonism[44].

Borderline personality disorder

Individual case reports and small studies have shown clozapine to be effective in the treatment of resistant cases of borderline personality disorder in reducing self-harm, aggressive behaviour and other associated symptoms[9–12].

Economic considerations

A full appraisal of the pharmacological benefits and costs associated with clozapine in the treatment of schizophrenia has been provided by Fitton and Benfield[45]. When in-patient and out-patient care, residential care, community-based services, drug therapy, and lost productivity and earnings, are all taken into consideration, it may be readily understood that schizophrenia places a major economical burden on society. The direct annual treatment cost of schizophrenia in the UK is estimated to be £1669 per person, comprising: hospital in-patient care (£572); other residential care (£662); out-patient visits (£56); day care (£228); community work, social work and GP fees (£63); depot injection clinic (£32); and drug therapy (£56, i.e. 3.4% of the total cost). Indirect costs associated with schizophrenia include morbidity, mortality, productive losses borne by relatives, and administration costs incurred by the community relating to criminal justice and social welfare. The overall cost of untreated aggression and violence within the health-care system and on society is difficult to estimate. Affective treatment of psychotic symptoms and associated aggression can bring down the total cost considerably.

Cautions and contra-indications

These include patients with myeloproliferative disorders, a history of toxic or idiosyncratic agranulocytosis or severe granulocytopaenia (with the exception of granulocytopaenia/agranulocytosis from previous chemotherapy). Clozapine is contra-indicated in patients with active liver disease, progressive liver disease and hepatic failure. Other contra-indications include severe CNS depression or comatose state, severe renal and cardiac disease, uncontrolled epilepsy, circulatory collapse, alcoholic/toxic psychosis and previous hypersensitivity to clozapine.

Side-effects

The most serious of clozapine's side-effects is agranulocytosis. Other important side-effects include postural hypotension and tachycardia, sedation, seizures, weight gain and rebound psychosis.

Clozapine can also cause:

- Nausea, vomiting and constipation.
- Elevation of liver enzymes (frequency up to 10%).
- Hypersalivation (frequency 12–40%).
- Confusion or delirium.
- Incontinence frequency/urgency, hesitancy, urinary retention, or impotence (6%).
- Benign hyperthermia (5–15%).

Isolated reports have been documented of clozapine-associated emergence of obsessive compulsive symptoms[46,47], priapism[48,49], allergic complications[50,51], pancreatitis[52], toxic hepatitis[53], elevation in creatinine kinase levels[54] and diabetes-like symptoms[55,56].

There have also been a handful of papers and case reports linking clozapine with raised triglyceride levels. Ghaeli and Dufresne[57] found that elevated serum triglycerides in four patients resolved when they were switched to risperidone. In two of these patients clozapine was re-introduced and again serum triglycerides increased. They called for serum triglyceride levels to be monitored in clozapine patients with additional cardiac risk factors. Dursun et al.[58] looked at cholesterol and related lipids in eight patients on clozapine treatment over 12 weeks. Serum triglyceride levels were found to increase, but not cholesterol levels.

Interactions

Drugs that cause CNS depression, if used concomitantly with clozapine, can increase both the frequency and the intensity of adverse effects such as drowsiness, sedation, dizziness and, possibly, respiratory depression. Ethanol and drugs like histamine blockers, benzodiazepines, opiate agonists, sedative-hypnotics and tricyclic antidepressants should be used with caution. Concomitant use of drugs known to cause bone marrow depression might increase the possibility of developing myelosuppressive effects. Clozapine has marked anticholinergic activity, and concurrent use with other anticholinergic drugs can increase side-effects, such as dry mouth, constipation, loss of accommodation and urinary retention. Carbamazepine, phenytoin and other cytochrome P-450 enzyme inducers can reduce clozapine plasma concentration. Clozapine in turn can increase the serum concentration of the following drugs: digoxin, heparin, phenytoin and warfarin. Drugs such as erythromycin, cimetidine, fluoxetine and fluvoxamine can inhibit cytochrome P-450 metabolism and can increase clozapine plasma concentration. Clozapine used concomitantly with other antihypertensive agents can increase the risk and severity of hypotension. Clozapine used in combination with lithium can increase the risk of developing seizures, confusion, dyskinesia and, possibly, neuroleptic malignant syndrome.

Conclusions

In terms of efficacy against conventional treatment-resistant schizophrenia, clozapine remains an unparalleled choice, although its general use is limited because of the risk of agranulocytosis.

References

1. Honigfield G. Effects of the Clozapine National Registry system on incidence of death related to agranulocytosis. *Psych Servs* 1996;47:52–6.
2. Walker AM, Lanza LL, Arellano F, Rothman KJ. Mortality in current and former users of clozapine. *Epidemiol* 1997;8:671–7.
3. Meltzer HY, *et al*. Reduction of suicidality during clozapine treatment of neuroleptic-resistant schizophrenia; impact on risk benefit assessment. *Am J Psych* 1995;152:183–90.
4. Kane J, Honigfield G, Singer J, *et al*. Clozapine for the treatment-resistant schizophrenic; a double blind comparison with chlorpromazine (Clozaril Collaborative Study). *Arch Gen Psych* 1988;45:789–96.
5. Kane J, Honigfield G, Singer J, *et al*. Clozapine for the treatment-resistant schizophrenic; results of a US multicenter trial. *Psychopharmacol* 1989;99:560–63.
6. Meltzer HY, *et al*. A prospective study of clozapine in treatment resistant schizophrenia patients. *Psychopharmacol* 1989;99(Suppl): 568–72.
7. Meltzer HY, *et al*. Dimensions of outcomes with clozapine. *Br J Psych* 1992;160(Suppl 17):46–53.
8. Change in clozapine monitoring requirements. *Phar J* 1995;May 6:254–612.
9. Frankenburge FR, Zanarini MC. *Comp Psych* 1993;34(6), Nov/Dec.
10. Steinert T, Schmidt-Michel PO, Kaschka WP. Considerable improvement in a case of obsessive–compulsive disorder in an emotionally unstable personality disorder, borderline type under treatment with clozapine: *Pharmacopsych* 1996;29(3):111–4.
11. Chengappa KN, Ebeling T, Kang JS, Levine J, Parepally H. Clozapine reduces severe self-mutilation and aggression in psychotic patients with borderline personality disorder. *J Clin Psych* 1999;60(7):477–84.
12. Benedetti F, Sforzini L, Colombo C, Maffei C, Smeraldi E. Low-dose clozapine in acute and continuation treatment of severe borderline personality disorder. *J Clin Psych* 1998;59(3):103–7.
13. The Bethlem & Maudsley NHS Trust Prescribing Guidelines, 1999.
14. Tandon R, Goldman R. Positive and negative symptoms during clopazine treatment in schizophrenia. *J Psych Res* 1993;Oct–Dec:341–7.
15. Lieberman JA, Safferman AZ, Pollack S, *et al*. Clinical effects of clozapine in chronic schizophrenia: response to treatment and predictors of outcome. *Am J Psych* 1994;151:1744–52.
16. Breier A, Buchanan RW, Kirkpatric B *et al*. Effects of clozapine on positive and negative symptoms in outpatients with schizophrenia. *Am J Psych* 1994;151:20.
17. Meltzer HY. Clozapine: is another view valid? *Am J Psych* 1995;152:821–5.
18. Singer and Law. A double blind comparison of clozapine and chlorpromazine in schizophrenia of acute symptomatology. *J Int Med* 1974; 2:433–5.
19. Gelenberg AJ, Doller JC. Clozapine versus chlorpromazine for the treatment of schizophrenia. *J Clin Psych* 1979;40(5):238–40.
20. Claghorn J, Honigfeld G, Abuzzahab FS Sr, Wang R, Steinbook R, Tuason V, Klerman G. The risk and benefits of clozapine versus chlorpromazine. *J Clin Psychopharmacol* 1987:7(6); 377–84.
21. Conley RR. Optimizing treatment with clozapine. *J Clin Psych* 1998;59(Suppl 3):44–8.
22. Lieberman JA. Maximizing clozapine therapy: managing side effects. *J Clin Psych* 1998;59 (Suppl 3):38–43.
23. Baldessarini RJ, Frankenburg FR. A novel antipsychotic agent. *New Engl J Med* 1991;324(11): 746–54.
24. UK clozapine study group. The safety and efficacy of clozapine in severe treatment-resistant schizophrenic patients in the UK. *Br J Psych* 1993;150–54.
25. Breier A. Buchanan RW. Kirkpatrick B. Davis OR. Irish D. Summerfelt A. Carpenter WT Jr. Effects of clozapine on positive and negative symptoms in outpatients with schizophrenia. *Am J Psych* 1994;151(1):20–6.

26. Meltzer HY, Burnett S, Bastani B, Ramirez LF. Effects of six months of clozapine treatment on the quality of life of chronic schizophrenic patients. *Hosp Comm Psych* 1990;41:892–7.
27. Avnon M. Rabinowitz J. Effectiveness of clozapine in hospitalized people with chronic schizophrenia. *Br J Psych* 1996;167(6):760–64.
28. Grace J, Bellus SB, Raulin ML, Herz MI, Priest BL, Brenner V, Donnelly K, Smith P, Gunn S. Long term impact of clozapine and psychosocial treatment on psychiatric symptoms and cognitive functioning. *Psych Servs* 1996;47(1): 41–5
29. Maier GJ. The impact of clozapine on 25 forensic patients. *Bull Am Acad Psych Law* 1992; 20(3):247–307.
30. Wilson WH. Clinical review of clozapine treatment in state hospital. *Hosp Commun Psych* 1992; 43(7):700–03.
31. Volavka J. The effects of clozapine on aggression and substance abuse in schizophrenic patients. *J Clin Psych* 1999; 60(Suppl 12):43–6.
32. Chiles JA, Davidson P, McBride D. Effects of clozapine in the use of seclusion and restraint in a state hospital. *Hosp Commun Psych*; 1994; 45(3):269–71
33. Ebrahim GM, Gibler B, Gacono CB, Hayes G. Patient response to clozapine in a forensic psychiatric hospital. *Hosp Comm Psych*; 1994;45(3): 271–3.
34. Buckley P, Bartell J, Donenwirth K, Lee S, Torigoe F, Schulz SC. Violence and schizophrenia: clozapine as specific anti-aggressive agent. *Bull Am Acad Psych Law* 1995;23(4):607–11.
35. Spivak B *et al*. Reduction of aggressiveness and impulsiveness during clozapine treatment in chronic treatment resistant schizophrenic patients. *Clin Neuropharmacol* 1997;20:442–6.
36. Green AL, *et al*. Clozapine for comorbid substance use disorder and schizophrenia; do patients with schizophrenia have a reward–deficiency syndrome that can be ameliorated by clozapine? *Harvard Rev Psych* 1999;6 (Mar–Apr):287–96.
37. Yovell Y, Opler LA. Clozapine reverses cocaine craving in a treatment resistant mentally ill chemical abuser: a case report and a hypothesis. *J Nerv Ment Dis* 1994;182(10):591–2.
38. Buckley P, Thompson P, Way L, Meltzer HY. Substance abuse among patients with treatment-resistant schizophrenia: characteristics and implications for clozapine therapy [see comments]. *Am J Psych* 1994;151(3):385–9.
39. Meltzer HY. Suicide and schizophrenia; clozapine and the InterSept study. *J Clin Psych* 1999; 60(Suppl 12):47–50.
40. Walker AM, Lanza LL. Mortality in current and former users of clozapine. *Epidemiology* 1997; 8(6):671–7.
41. Suppes T, Phillips KA, Judd CR. Clozapine treatment of nonpsychotic rapid cycling bipolar disorder: a report of three cases. *Biol Psych* 1994;36(5):338–40.
42. Zarate CA Jr, Tohen M, Baldessarini RJ. Clozapine in severe mood disorder. *J Clin Psych* 1995; 56(9):411–7.
43. McElroy SL. Clozapine in the treatment of psychotic mood disorders, schizo-effective disorder and schizophrenia. *J Clin Psych* 1991;52: 411–4.
44. The Parkinson's Study Group. Low dose clozapine for the treatment of drug induced psychosis in Parkinson's disease. *New Engl J Med* 1999; 340:757–63
45. Fitton A. Benfield P. Clozapine and its pharmacoeconomic benefits in the treatment of schizophrenia. *Pharm Econ* 1993;(August):31–56.
46. Baker RW, Chengappa KN, Baird JW, Steingard S, Christ MA, Schooler NR. Emergence of obsessive compulsive symptoms during treatment with clozapine [see Comments]. *J Clin Psych* 1992;53(12):439–42.
47. Patil VJ. Development of transient obsessive–compulsive symptoms during treatment with clozapine. *Am J Psych* 1992;149:272.
48. Zeilger J, Behar D. Clozapine induced priapism. *Am J Psych* 1992;149:272–3.
49. Rosen SL, Hanno PM. Clozapine induced priapism. *J Urol* 1992;148(Sept):876–7.
50. Stoppe G. Life threatening allergic reaction to clozapine. *Br J Psych* 1992;161:259–61.
51. Wickert WA, Campbell NR, Martin L. Acute severe adverse clozapine reaction resembling systemic lupus erythematosus [Letter]. *Postgrad Med J* 1994;70(830):940–41.
52. Martin A. Acute pancreatitis associated with clozapine use [Letter]. *Am J Psych* 1992;149: 714.
53. Kellner M, Wiedemann K, Krieg JC, Berg PA. Toxic hepatitis by clozapine treatment [Letter] [see Comments]. *Am J Psych* 1993;150(6):985–6.
54. Kirson JL. Severe elevation in serum creatinine kinase associated with clozapine [Letter]. *J Clin Psychopharm* 1995;15(4):287–8.
55. Koval MS. Diabetic ketoacidosis associated with clozapine treatment. *Am J Psych* 1994;151: 1520–21.

56. Kamran A. Severe hyperglycaemia with high doses of clozapine. *Am J Psych* 1994;151:1395.
57. Ghaeli P, Dufresne RL. Elevated serum triglycerides with clozapine resolved with risperidone in four patients. *Pharmacother* 1999;19(9):1099–101.
58. Dursun SM, Szemis A, Andrews H, Reveley MA. The effects of clozapine on levels of total cholesterol and related lipids in serum of patients with schizophrenia: a prospective study. *J Psych Neurosci* 1999;24(5):453–5.

Chapter 8
Focus on Risperidone

Dr Ben Green

Summary

Risperidone is an antipsychotic available worldwide since the early 1990s. It has been characterised as atypical, but shares some of the extrapyramidal side effect profile of the earlier antipsychotics, particularly at higher doses.

Introduction

Risperidone has been developed by Janssen-Cilag. It is a novel antipsychotic with dopaminergic and serotonergic effects. Risperidone is available in tablet and liquid form. A depot formulation is available.

The main pharmacological activities of risperidone include serotonin 5-HT$_2$ receptor blockade and dopamine D$_2$ antagonism[39]. After oral administration of 1 mg of risperidone 5-HT$_2$ receptor occupancy is about 60% and D$_2$ dopamine receptor occupancy in the striatum is about 50%[43]. In common with other antipsychotics, risperidone enhances prolactin release, but some central effects such as catalepsy and blockade of motor activity occur at high doses only. Risperidone is 4–10 times less potent than the conventional antipsychotic haloperidol as a central D$_2$ antagonist in rats. Interaction with dopamine D1 receptors occurs only at very high concentrations. The pharmacological profile of risperidone includes interaction with histamine H$_1$ and alpha-adrenergic receptors but the compound does not interact significantly with cholinergic receptors.

The drug has good activity against various symptoms and signs associated with schizophrenia[36]. Compared to conventional antipsychotics such as haloperidol risperidone produces some significantly better results according to Positive and Negative Syndrome Scale (PANSS) scores. Marder et al.'s study[36] factor analysed the PANSS scores and produced five dimensions; negative symptoms, positive symptoms, disorganized thought, uncontrolled hostility/excitement, and anxiety/depression. The study looked at 513 patients in two double-blind trials. Symptom reductions in PANSS factor scores from baseline to treatment at weeks 6 and 8 were significantly greater in patients receiving 6–16 mg/day of risperidone than in patients receiving placebo or haloperidol.

The advantages of risperidone were greatest for negative symptoms, uncontrolled hostility/excitement, and anxiety/depression.

Meta-analysis from available randomised, double-masked, comparative trials of risperidone and haloperidol in patients with schizophrenia treated for at least 4 weeks at recommended doses[14]. Six out of nine trials met all criteria for inclusion in the meta-analysis which showed that in patients with chronic schizophrenia, risperidone therapy is associated with significantly higher response rates, significantly less prescribing of anticholinergic medication, and significantly lower treatment dropout rates than haloperidol.

Dosage Regime

In adults the suggested initial dose schedule for risperidone is to titrate doses upward from 1 mg twice daily, to 2 mg b.d. the next day and 3 mg b.d. the day after to achieve a dose of 4–6 mg daily. However, there has been recent work recommending a less rapid titration (over 6 days to a week) and that the dose increments consist of 0.5–2 mg/day[34]. The starting dose in the elderly is 0.5 mg b.d. with 0.5 mg increments to 2 mg b.d.

The conventional dosing regime is twice daily, although there has been recent interest in a once-daily regime. A recent double-blind 6-week study of 211 patients with acute exacerbation were randomly assigned to receive risperidone at 8mg once daily or 4mg twice daily. The study demonstrated little clinical difference between 8mg given once daily and 4 mg given twice daily[42].

In terms of switching patients over from conventional antipsychotics to risperidone about sixty per cent of patients can have their current neuroleptics stopped and risperidone started immediately together with a gradual withdrawal of anticholinergic treatments[30]. This strategy is understandably more successful for who previously received conventional antipsychotics as depot medication.

Nyberg et al.[44] have suggested 4 mg/day as the best minimal dosage regime based on PET receptor occupancy studies. They comment that treatment with risperidone, 6 mg/day, is likely to induce unnecessarily high D_2 receptor occupancy, with a consequent extrapyramidal side effects. They found that high 5-HT_{2A} receptor occupancy did not prevent extrapyramidal side effects completely. The authors previously suggested an optimal interval for D_2 receptor occupancy of 70–80%. To achieve this, they suggested risperidone, 4 mg/day, as a suitable initial dose for antipsychotic effect with a minimal risk of extrapyramidal side effects in most patients.

Structure

Risperidone (R64 766) is a benzisoxazole derivative whose molecular formula is $C_{23}H_{27}FN_4O_2$. Figure 8.1 is a diagram of the risperidone molecule.

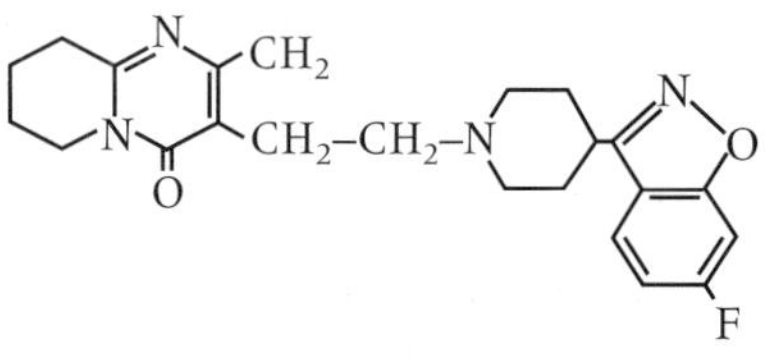

Figure 8.1: *The risperidone molecule.*

Binding Profile

Table 8.1, derived from Schotte et al.[48], shows the *in vitro* receptor binding profile for risperidone. In the table K_i indicates the drug concentration needed to inhibit binding of a ligand selective for a receptor by 50%. A low K_i indicates a high affinity.

It is the Serotonin 5-HT_{2A} and Dopamine D_2 receptor occupancy that seem to provide the therapeutic effects of risperidone. In vivo PET studies have found that the Serotonin 5-HT_{2A} and Dopamine D_2 receptor occupancy rates are 60% in the neocortex and 50% in the striatum for the respective receptor types[43]. The Serotonin 5-HT_{2A} binding in the cortex disinhibits the mesocortical dopamine system, resulting in an increase in dopamine transmission in this pathway and is thought to account for the clinical efficacy against negative and affective symptoms.

A tantalizing study by Tarazi et al.[59] looked at long-term receptor status in rats treated with quetaipine, risperidone and olanzapine. Antipsychotic effects of olanzapine and risperidone are partly mediated by D_2 receptors in the medial prefrontal cortex, nucleus accumbens, or hippocampus, and perhaps D_4 receptors in caudate-putamen, nucleus accumbens, or hippocampus, but not in cerebral cortex. Selective up-regulation of D_2 receptors by olanzapine and risperidone in caudate-putamen may reflect their ability to induce some extrapyramidal effects. They found an inability of quetiapine to alter dopamine receptors and suggested that nondopaminergic mechanisms were responsible for its antipsychotic effects (which merits replication and further study).

Table 8.1:

Receptor Type	Animal Brain		Cloned Human Receptors	
	Risperidone K_i (nM)	Haloperidol K_i (nM)	Risperidone K_i (nM)	Haloperidol K_i (nM)
Serotonin 5-HT_{2A}	0.16	25	0.52	200
Dopamine D_2	3.3	1.4	5.9	2.2
Dopamine D_1	620	270	-	-
Noradrenaline a_1	2.3	19	-	-
Noradrenaline a_2	7.5	>5000	Range 8.5–23	Range 480–1130
Histamine H_1	2.6	730	27	790
Acetylcholine muscarinic	>5000	4670	-	-

Clinical Indications and Efficacy

As far as the manufacturers are concerned risperidone is indicated for acute and chronic schizophrenic psychoses and other psychotic conditions with positive and negative symptoms. It is also indicated for affective symptoms associated with schizophrenia[2]. There is quite ample evidence of its efficacy in schizophrenia[54]. Schizoaffective disorder[65] also appears to be a promising area for the prescription of risperidone. In their study 95 patients with DSM-IV schizoaffective disorder completed a six week open label trial of the drug and improved in terms of their psychosis and affective symptomatology.

There is some evidence that risperidone is useful to some extent in reducing aggression in schizophrenia[11], although possibly not more effectively than typical antipsychotics[5].

Delusions of infestation appear responsive in small series studies[16].

There is some evidence for its usefulness as an adjunctive therapy in acute bipolar affective disorder in outpatients[21] and in bipolar disorder when followed up over a six-month period[22]. It has been postulated that there is dopaminergic mediation as well as a serotonergic mediation for some obsessive and related disorders e.g. Tourette's syndrome. Risperidone has therefore also been used to augment SSRIs in obsessive compulsive disorder[47,57]. In Saxena *et al.*'s study about eighty per cent of patients improved within three weeks of the addition of risperidone. In a series of 22 patients risperidone was found to be effective in 58%[12]. In affective psychoses, risperidone is probably not useful as a *single* therapeutic agent, that is to say it does not seem to replace an antipsychotic/antidepressant combination[41].

Risperidone has been found useful in adolescent schizophrenia[1] and in children with autistic/pervasive developmental disorders[17,38]. Tourette's syndrome appears to be treatable with risperidone and somewhat superior to earlier treatments such as pimozide. Bruggeman's 2001 study[69] showed that risperidone produced significant improvement of tics using the Tourette's Symptom Severity Scale (TSSS). At the end of the study, 54% (14/26) of the risperidone patients and 38% (9/24) of the pimozide patients had only very mild or no symptoms on the global severity rating of the TSSS

There has been considerable interest and study of its use in the elderly. There has been documented beneficial use in dementia with persistent vocalisations[32], and in demented people with Parkinson's[67]. Katz *et al.*[26] found that 1 mg/day was useful in controlling aggression in severe dementia.

There is ample study and anecdotal evidence for the use of risperidone in liaison psychiatry, uses include delirium[19,53] and HIV-related psychotic disorders[52].

Pharmacokinetics

Risperidone is rapidly and very well absorbed after administration orally; less than 1% is excreted unchanged in the faeces[24]. Risperidone is 90% plasma protein bound[8]. The principal metabolite is 9-hydroxyrisperidone. Hydroxylation of risperidone is subject to the same genetic CYP2D6-related polymorphism as for debrisoquine and dextromethorphan. In poor metabolizers the half-life of risperidone was about 20 hours compared with about 3 hours in extensive metabolizers[25]. However, because the pharmacology of 9-hydroxyrisperidone is very similar to that of risperidone, the half-life for the 'active moiety' (risperidone +9-hydroxyrisperidone) was found to be about 20 hours in poor metabolizers. Risperidone exhibits linear elimination kinetics. Steady state is reached within 1 day for risperidone and within 5 days for the active fraction.

Health Economics

There has been considerable debate about the direct medication costs and the cost efficacy of novel antipsychotics such as risperidone. There are health economic studies that indicate reduced indirect costs associated with poor compliance, such as repeated acute ward admissions, but also perhaps a shift in resources towards community care (day hospital places and the like). Viale *et al.*[64] investigated costs associated with risperidone and found days in acute care inpatient facilities were reduced by 26 per cent, and days in residential treatment were reduced by 57 per cent. These reductions were accompanied by an increase in the use of lower-cost services, such as community and day hospital treatment.

Risperidone and other atypical antipsychotics appear to promote a higher quality of life compared to conventional antipsychotics. Physical well being, social life and everyday life have also been rated higher in a comparative study using risperidone[18]. In one evaluation, compared to haloperidol, a conventional antipsychotic, risperidone-treated patients obtained more than twice as many quality-adjusted years as haloperidol patients and in addition risperidone was found to be cost-effective[13]. A US evaluation of costs, including indirect ones came up with figures for treatment with haloperidol and risperidone[28]. A robust decision-analytic model of schizophrenia suggested that the overall 1997 cost of treating a patient with risperidone would be $11 772.00 per year compared with $13 622.00 per year for haloperidol and that the cost per response is even more favourable for risperidone; $14 599.00 versus $23 040.00.

Guidelines issued by the Australian Pharmaceutical Benefits Advisory Committee have been used to construct a model for comparing the cost-effectiveness of risperidone and haloperidol over a 2-year period in patients with chronic schizophrenia[15]. Cost-effectiveness was determined by using decision-analytic modelling. The analyses included all significant direct costs (i.e., hospital costs; outpatient costs; and the cost of drugs, the services of health care professionals, and government-subsidised hostel accommodation). The cost for a given outcome was the sum of costs for all scenarios leading to that outcome. Cost-effectiveness was expressed as the total cost per favourable outcome, i.e. where the patient was responding to treatment at the end of the 2-year period. The probability of a patient experiencing a favourable outcome at the end of 2 years was 78.9% for risperidone versus 58.9% for haloperidol. The total cost of treatment for 2 years was $15 549.00 for risperidone versus $18 332.00 for haloperidol. The expected cost per favourable outcome was $19 709.00 for risperidone and $31 104.00 for haloperidol. Risperidone was more cost-effective than haloperidol and therefore was 'dominant' in pharmacoeconomic terms because it produced a higher proportion of favourable outcomes at lower cost.

A more recent study of nearly 800 patients comparing risperidone and olanzapine found swifter discharges and lower drug costs associated with risperidone[27].

Adverse effects

Common side effects include insomnia (about 8% of patients), weight gain, agitation, anxiety and headache. Less frequent side effects include somnolence, tiredness, dizziness, poor concentration, nausea, and dysfunctions of erection, ejaculation and orgasm.

Orthostatic hypotension can occur particularly initially. Prolactin rises can induce galactorrhoea and gynaecomastia along with disturbances of the menstrual cycle and amenorrhoea[29]. Prolactin rises are also documented in males[37].

Risperidone appears to have less potential for causing EPS than conventional antipsychotics and as such may be more suitable as a maintenance antipsychotic than conventional dopamine-blockers[31]. In a study completed by over two hundred chronic schizophrenic patients by Simpson & Lindenmayer[50] the severity of EPS in a risperidone treated group as measured by the Extrapyramidal Symptom Rating Scale (ESRS) score did not differ significantly differ from placebo group. There was a linear relationship between mean change scores and increasing risperidone dose on 4 of the 12 ESRS subscales. However, even at 16 mg/day of risperidone, mean change scores were lower than in a group treated with haloperidol group. A linear relationship between increasing risperidone dose and use of antiparkinsonian medications was also apparent.

In a study of more than a hundred elderly patients, often with co-morbid medical conditions risperidone was found to be a safe and effective antipsychotic[68]. In this study there were adverse events in 32% of the patients. These adverse events included hypotension (29%), extrapyramidal effects (11%), symptomatic orthostasis (10%), cardiac arrest (1.6%) with fatality (0.8%), and delirium (1.6%).

There are several reports of neuroleptic malignant syndrome with risperidone[4,7,23,46,51]. There is at least one recent report associating a year's exposure to risperidone with tardive dyskinesia, although this was in a patient who had previously been exposed to classical antipsychotics[49]. There have been reports of priapism associated with risperidone[60]. There is at least one case report of risperidone causing sudden cardiac death[45]. Annual adverse event monitoring in the UK has shown that the relative risk with risperidone compared to other antipsychotics is decreased[61]. Annual reporting rates for tardive dyskinesia were 0.0006% of patients and neuroleptic malignant syndrome 0.017%. EPS reports were made for 0.2% of patients. It is unlikely though that all adverse events are reported, and these probably represent an underestimate of the true incidence.

A variant tardive abnormal movement, rabbit syndrome, has been described with risperidone[33]. Rabbit syndrome is a rare side effect of chronic neuroleptic administration characterized by rapid, fine, rhythmic movements of the mouth along a vertical axis.

Overdoses of up to 360 mg have been reported. Problems include sedation, tachycardia, hypotension and EPS. QT prolongation may occur on ECG. One of the first overdoses with risperidone was noted in 1993. ECG abnormalities were recorded, but there was no fatality[10]. Nevertheless, fatalities have been reported[56].

No teratogenic effect has been yet noted, but caution should be exercised before prescribing in pregnancy. Risperidone is excreted in milk in animal studies. Women receiving risperidone should not therefore breast feed.

Interactions

There may be interactions with carbamazepine, which decreases the plasma levels of the antipsychotic fraction of risperidone. Similar drugs that induce hepatic enzymes may have the same effect. Phenothiazines, tricyclic antidepressants, fluoxetine, haloperidol and some beta blockers can increase plasma concentrations of risperidone.

Co-administration of paroxetine may increase plasma levels of risperidone and its active moiety 9-OH-risperidone by as much as 45%[55]

Comparison with other antipsychotics

Extrapyramidal side effects, hyperprolactinemia, and sexual dysfunction are significantly more frequent with risperidone than olanzapine[62]. Weight gain though is more common with olanzapine than risperidone[20]. In their four-month study of 100 patients, with fifty treated with either risperidone or olanzapine in each group, mean weight gain with olanzapine was 2 kg, with no mean weight gain in risperidone patients.

Patients who are treatment resistant as conventionally defined may probably be better treated with clozapine. However there is at least one recent study that suggests that a trial of risperidone may be worthwhile in conventional antipsychotic treatment resistance[6]. There appears to be little benefit to switching patients non-responsive to clozapine to risperidone[58]. Clozapine is more effective than risperidone at reducing positive symptoms in resistant patients and is less likely to disturb the prolactin system[9]. Other recent studies such as that of Azorin et al.[3] indicate the superiority of clozapine in chronic schizophrenia and the reduced likelihood of extrapyramidal side effects with clozapine.

Risperidone has different intracerebral effects compared to haloperidol as measured by cerebral blood flow. Positron emission tomography imaging by Miller et al.[40] demonstrated that haloperidol is associated with a significantly greater increase in regional cerebral blood flow in the left putamen and posterior cingulate, and a significantly reduced blood flow in frontal regions compared to risperidone. Risperidone decreased cerebral blood flow in the cerebellum bilaterally compared to haloperidol.

Compared to other second generation antipsychotics risperidone has low to moderate tendencies to cause weight gain. It is less likely to cause weight gain than olanzapine or clozapine[66].

Malla et al.[35] compared risperidone and first generation antipsychotics in a cohort of 126 patients in which there were two groups of 19 first-episode DSM-III-R/DSM-IV schizophrenia patients matched for age, gender, length of illness, and length of treatment and treated with either a typical antipsychotic or risperidone for a minimum of 1 year. The groups were compared on a number of outcome measures. Treatment allocation was not random, and patients were judged to be compliant with medication. Six patients (31.6%) from the typical antipsychotic group were admitted to the hospital within the first year following the index admission compared with 1 patient (5.3%) in the risperidone group (admitted at month 14). Patients in the risperidone group showed a statistically significantly lower length of first hospitalization ($p < .01$), utilization of inpatient beds during the course of treatment ($p < .001$), and use of anticholinergic medication ($p < .05$). There were no statistically significant differences in symptom levels, either during the course of treatment or at follow-up; in the use of antidepressant, anxiolytic, or mood-stabilizing drugs; or in changes in living circumstances or employment. The authors concluded that there was equal long-term efficacy of typical antipsychotics and risperidone, but a possible advantage for risperidone in decreased use of services and also less use of concomitant anticholinergic drugs.

Conclusion

Risperidone is one of a new generation of antipsychotic drugs with relatively fewer side effects and equal efficacy for florid 'positive' symptoms compared to first generation antipsychotics such as chlorpromazine. The additional serotonergic actions of risperidone appear to deliver further efficacy against 'negative' and affective symptoms of schizophrenia. There are however differences in the side effect profiles of the new antipsychotics and in some instances risperidone performs less well than others especially where higher doses are involved, inducing extrapyramidal side effects. Despite their higher direct costs some antipsychotics, particularly risperidone, have interesting economic arguments in their favour compared to earlier antipsychotics.

References

1. Armenteros JL, Whitaker AH, Welikson M, Stedge J, Gorman J (1997). Risperidone in adolescents with schizophrenia: an open pilot study. *J Am Acad Child Adolesc Psychiatry*, 36(5): 694–700.
2. Association of British Pharmaceutical Industries (1998). ABPI Compendium of Data Sheets. Summaries of Product Characteristics 1998–99. London, ABPI.
3. Azorin JM, Spiegel R, Remington G, Vanelle JM, Pere JJ, Giguere M, Bourdeix I (2001). A double-blind comparative study of clozapine and risperidone in the management of severe chronic schizophrenia. *American Journal of Psychiatry*, 158(8):1305–13, 2001 Aug.
4. Bajjoka I, Patel T, O'Sullivan T (1997) Risperidone-induced neuroleptic malignant syndrome. *Ann. Emerg. Med*, 30(5): 698–700.
5. Beck NC, *et al*. (1997). Risperidone in the management of violent, treatment-resistant schizophrenics hospitalized in a maximum security forensic facility. *Am. Acad. Psychiatry Law*, 25(4): 461–8.
6. Bondolfi *et al*. (1998). Risperidone versus clozapine in treatment-resistant chronic schizophrenia: a randomized double-blind study. The Risperidone Study Group. *Am. J. Psychiatry*, 155(4): 499–504.
7. Bonwick RJ, Hopwood MJ, Morris PL (1996). Neuroleptic malignant syndrome and risperidone: a case report. *Aust. N.Z.J. Psychiatry*, 30(3): 419–21.
8. Borison R (1994). Risperidone: pharmacokinetics. *J. Clin. Psychiatry Monograph*, 12(2):46–48.
9. Breier AF, Malhotra AK, Su TP, *et al*. (1999). Clozapine and risperidone in chronic schizophrenia: effects on symptoms, parkinsonian side effects, and neuroendocrine response. *Am J Psychiatry*, 156:2, 294–8.
10. Brown K (1993). Overdose of risperidone. *Ann. Emerg. Med*, 22(12):1908–10.
11. Buckley F, *et al*. (1997). Aggression and schizophrenia: efficacy of risperidone. *J. Am. Acad. Psychiatry Law*, 25(2): 173–81.
12. Bruun RD, Budman CL (1996). Risperidone as a treatment for Tourette's syndrome. *J. Clin. Psychiatry*, 57(1): 29–31.
13. Chouinard G, Albright PS (1997). Economic and health state utility determinations for schizophrenic patients treated with risperidone or haloperidol. *J. Clin. Psychopharmacol.*, 17(4): 298–307.
14. Davies A, *et al*. (1998). Risperidone versus haloperidol: I. Meta-analysis of efficacy and safety. *Clin. Ther*, 20(1):58–71.
15. Davies A, *et al*. (1998). Risperidone versus haloperidol: II. Cost-effectiveness. *Clin. Ther.*, 20(1): 196–213.
16. De-Leon OA, Furmaga KM, Canterbury AL, Bailey LG (1997). Risperidone in the treatment of delusions of infestation. *Int. J. Psychiatry Med.*, 27(4): 403–9.
17. Findling RL, Maxwell K, Wiznitzer M (1997). An open clinical trial of risperidone monotherapy in young children with autistic disorder. *Psychopharmacol. Bull.*, 33(1): 155–9.
18. Franz M, Lis S, Pluddemann K, Gallhofer B (1997). Conventional versus atypical neuroleptics: subjective quality of life in schizophrenic patients. *Br J Psychiatry*, 170: 422–5.
19. Furmaga KM, *et al*. (1997). Psychosis in medical conditions: response to risperidone. *Gen. Hosp. Psychiatry*, 19(3): 223–8.
20. Ganguli R, Brar JS, Ayrton Z (2001). Weight gain over 4 months in schizophrenia patients: a

comparison of olanzapine and risperidone. *Schizophrenia Research*, 49(3):261–7, 2001 Apr 30.
21. Ghaemi SN, Sachs GS, Baldassano CF, Truman CJ (1997). Acute treatment of bipolar disorder with adjunctive risperidone in outpatients. *Can. J. Psychiatry*, 42(2):196–9.
22. Ghaemi SN, Sachs GS (1997). Long-term risperidone treatment in bipolar disorder: 6-month follow up. *Int-Clin-Psychopharmacol.*, 12(6):333–8.
23. Gleason PP, Conigliaro RL (1997). Neuroleptic malignant syndrome with risperidone. *Pharmacotherapy*, 17(3):617–21.
24. Heykants J, Huang ML, Mannens G, Meuldermans W, Snoeck E, Van Beijsterveldt L, Van Peer A, Woestenborghs R (1994). The pharmacokinetics of risperidone in humans: a summary. *J. Clin. Psychiatry*, 55 Suppl: 13–7, May 1994.
25. Huang ML, et al. (1993). Pharmacokinetics of the novel antipsychotic agent risperidone and the prolactin response in healthy subjects. *Clin. Pharmacol. Ther.*, 54(3):257–68.
26. Katz IR, Jeste DV, Mintzer JE, et al. (1999). Comparison of risperidone and placebo for psychosis and behavioral disturbances associated with dementia: a randomized, double-blind trial. Risperidone Study Group. *J. Clin. Psychiatry*, 60:2,107–15.
27. Kelly DL, Nelson MW, Love RC, Yu Y, Conley RR (2001). Comparison of discharge rates and drug costs for patients with schizophrenia treated with risperidone or olanzapine. *Psychiatric Services*, 52(5):676–8, 2001 May.
28. Keks NA (1997). Impact of newer antipsychotics on outcomes in schizophrenia. *Clin. Ther.*, 19(1):148–58; discussion 126–7.
29. Kim YK, Kim L, Lee MS (1999). Risperidone and associated amenorrhea: a report of 5 cases. *J Clin Psychiatry*, 60:5, 315–7.
30. Kirov GK, Murray RM, Seth RV, Feeney S (1997). Observations on switching patients with schizophrenia to risperidone treatment. Risperidone Switching Study Group. *Acta. Psychiatr. Scand.*, 95(5):439–43.
31. Kopala LC, Good KP, Honer WG (1997). Extrapyramidal signs and clinical symptoms in first-episode schizophrenia: response to low-dose risperidone. *J. Clin. Psychopharmacol.*, 17(4):308–13.
32. Kopala LC, Honer WG (1997). The use of risperidone in severely demented patients with persistent vocalizations. *Int. J. Geriatr. Psychiatry*, 12(1):73–7.
33. Levin T & Heresco Levy U (1999). Risperidone-induced rabbit syndrome: an unusual movement disorder caused by an atypical antipsychotic. *Eur Neuropsychopharmacol*, 9:1–2, 137–9.
34. Luchins DJ, Klass D, Hanrahan P, Malan R, Harris J (1998). Alteration in the recommended dosing schedule for risperidone. *Am. J. Psychiatry*, 155(3): 365–6.
35. Malla AK, Norman RM, Scholten DJ, Zirul S, Kotteda V (2001). A comparison of long-term outcome in first-episode schizophrenia following treatment with risperidone or a typical antipsychotic. *Journal of Clinical Psychiatry*, 62(3):179–84, 2001 Mar.
36. Marder SR, Davis JM, Chouinard G (1997). The effects of risperidone on the five dimensions of schizophrenia derived by factor analysis: combined results of the North American trials. *J. Clin. Psychiatry*, 58(12): 538–46.
37. Markianos M, Hatzimanolis J, Lykouras L (1999). Gonadal axis hormones in male schizophrenic patients during treatment with haloperidol and after switch to risperidone. *Psychopharmacology Berl*, 143:3, 270–2.
38. McDougle CJ, et al. (1997). Risperidone treatment of children and adolescents with pervasive developmental disorders: a prospective open-label study. *J. Am. Acad. Child Adolesc. Psychiatry*, 36(5): 685–93.
39. Megens AA (1994). Survey on the pharmacodynamics of the new antipsychotic risperidone. *Psychopharmacology Berl*, 114(1): 9–23.
40. Miller DD, Andreasen NC, O,Leary DS, Watkins GL, Boles Ponto LL, Hichwa RD (2001). Comparison of the effects of risperidone and haloperidol on regional cerebral blood flow in schizophrenia. *Biological Psychiatry*, 49(8):704–15, 2001 Apr 15.
41. Muller–Siecheneder F, Muller MJ, Hillert A, Szegedi A, Wetzel H (1998). Risperidone versus haloperidol and amitriptyline in the treatment of patients with a combined psychotic and depressive syndrome. *J. Clin. Psychopharmacol.*, 18(2): 111–20.
42. Nair NP (1998). Therapeutic equivalence of risperidone given once daily and twice daily in patients with schizophrenia. The Risperidone Study Group. *J. Clin. Psychopharmacol.*, 18(2): 103–10.
43. Nyberg S, et al. (1993). 5-HT2 and D_2 dopamine receptor occupancy in the living human brain. A PET study with risperidone. *Psychopharmacology Berl*, 110(3): 265–72.
44. Nyberg S, Eriksson B, Oxenstierna G, Halldin C, Farde L (1999). Suggested minimal effective

dose of risperidone based on PET-measured D$_2$ and 5-HT2A receptor occupancy in schizophrenic patients. *Am J Psychiatry*, 156:6, 869–75.
45. Ravin DS, Levenson JW (1997). Fatal cardiac event following initiation of risperidone therapy. *Ann. Pharmacother.*, 31(7–8): 867–70.
46. Robb AS, Chang W, Lee HK, Cook MS (2000). Case study. Risperidone-Induced neuroleptic malignant syndrome in an adolescent. *Journal of Child & Adolescent Psychopharmacology*. 10(4): 327–30, 2000 Winter.
47. Saxena S, Wang D, Bystritsky A, Baxter LR (1996). Risperidone augmentation of SRI treatment for refractory obsessive-compulsive disorder. *J. Clin. Psychiatry*, 57(7):303–6.
48. Schotte A, Janssen PFM, Gommeren W (1996). Risperdine compared with new and reference antipsychotic drugs: *in vitro* and *in vivo* receptor binding. *Psychpharmacol.*, 124:57–73.
49. Silberbauer C (1998). Risperidone-induced tardive dyskinesia. *Pharmacopsychiatry*, 31(2):68–9.
50. Simpson GM, Lindenmayer JP (1997). Extrapyramidal symptoms in patients treated with risperidone. *J. Clin. Psychopharmacol.*, 17(3): 194–201.
51. Singer S, Richards C, Boland RJ (1995). Two cases of risperidone-induced neuroleptic malignant syndrome [letter]. *Am. J. Psychiatry*, 152(8):1234.
52. Singh AN, Golledge H, Catalan J (1997). Treatment of HIV-related psychotic disorders with risperidone: a series of 21 cases. *J. Psychosom. Res.*, 42(5): 489–93.
53. Sipahimalani A, Masand PS (1997). Use of risperidone in delirium: case reports. *Ann-Clin-Psychiatry*, 9(2): 105–7.
54. Song F (1997). Risperidone in the treatment of schizophrenia: a meta-analysis of randomized controlled trials. *J. Psychopharmacol. Oxf.*, 11(1): 65–71.
55. Spina E, Avenoso A, Facciola G, Scordo MG (2001). Ancione M. Madia A. Plasma concentrations of risperidone and 9-hydroxyrisperidone during combined treatment with paroxetine. *Therapeutic Drug Monitoring*, 23(3):223–7, 2001 Jun.
56. Springfield AC, Bodiford E (1996). An overdose of risperidone. *J. Anal. Toxicol.*, 20(3):202–3.
57. Stein DJ, Bouwer C, Hawkridge S, Emsley RA (1997). Risperidone augmentation of serotonin reuptake inhibitors in obsessive–compulsive and related disorders. *J. Clin. Psychiatry*, 58(3): 119–22.
58. Still DJ, *et al.* (1996). Effects of switching inpatients with treatment-resistant schizophrenia from clozapine to risperidone. *Psychiatr. Serv.*, 47(12): 1382–4.
59. Tarazi FI, Zhang K, Baldessarini RJ (2001). Long-term effects of olanzapine, risperidone, and quetiapine on dopamine receptor types in regions of rat brain: implications for antipsychotic drug treatment. *Journal of Pharmacology & Experimental Therapeutics*, 297(2):711–7, 2001 May.
60. Tekell JL, Smith EA, Silva JA (1995). Prolonged erection associated with risperidone treatment [letter]. *Am. J. Psychiatry*, 152(7): 1097.
61. Tooley PJH, Zuiderwijk P (1997). Drug safety: Experience with risperidone. *Advances in Therapy*, Vol. 14(5):262–266.
62. Tran PV, *et al.* (1997). Double-blind comparison of olanzapine versus risperidone in the treatment of schizophrenia and other psychotic disorders. *J. Clin. Psychopharmacol.*, 17(5): 407–18.
63. Umbricht D, Kane JM (1996). Medical complications of new antipsychotic drugs. *Schizophr. Bull.*, 22(3): 475–83.
64. Viale G, *et al.* (1997). Impact of risperidone on the use of mental health care resources. *Psychiatr. Serv.*, 48(9): 1153–9.
65. Vieta E, Herraiz M, Fernandez A, Gasto C, Benabarre A, Colom F, Martinez-Aran A, Reinares M (2001). Efficacy and safety of risperidone in the treatment of schizoaffective disorder: initial results from a large, multicenter surveillance study. Group for the Study of Risperidone in Affective Disorders (GSRAD). *Journal of Clinical Psychiatry*, 62(8):623–30, 2001 Aug.
66. Wirshing DA, Wirshing WC, Kysar L, *et al.* (1999). Novel antipsychotics: comparison of weight gain liabilities. *J Clin Psychiatry*, 60(6): 358–63, 1999 Jun.
67. Workman RH, *et al.* (1998). The use of risperidone for psychosis and agitation in demented patients with Parkinson's disease. *J. Neuropsychiatry Clin. Neurosci.*, 9(4): 594–7.
68. Zarate C, *et al.* (1997). Risperidone in the elderly: a pharmacoepidemiologic study. *J. Clin. Psychiatry*, 58(7): 311–7.
69. Bruggeman R, van der Linden C, Buitelaar JK, Gericke GS, Hawkridge SM, Temlett JA. Risperidone versus pimozide in Tourette's disorder: a comparative double-blind parallel-group study. *Journal of Clinical Psychiarty*, 62(1): 50–6, 2001.

Chapter 9
Focus on Olanzapine

Dr Ben Green

Summary

Olanzapine* is a novel antipsychotic agent of the theinobenzodiazepine class developed by Eli Lilly & Co. It has a pleotrophic pharmacology and affects the dopaminergic, serotonergic, muscarinic and adrenergic systems. The therapeutic advantage of recent antipsychotics (so-called atypical antipsychotics) has been attributed to additional serotonergic effects. Clinical studies and trials suggest that olanzapine is comparable or superior to haloperidol and may be superior to risperidone in terms of efficacy and side-effect profiles.

The starting dose of olanzapine is a single dose of 10 mg. The drug reaches peak plasma levels in 5–8 hours, and has a half-life of about 35 hours depending on metabolism. The recommended maximum dose is 20 mg daily, but higher doses have been employed.

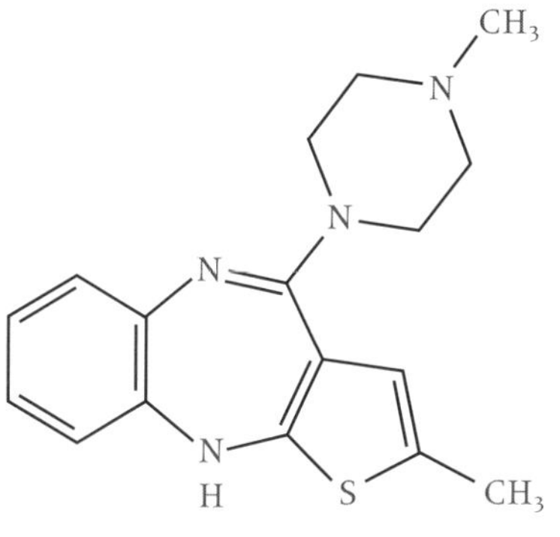

Figure 9.1: *Olanzapine chemical structure*[31].

Abnormalities of the QTc interval on ECG are unlikely to occur[8]. The most common side-effects are somnolence and weight gain. About 40% of patients in clinical trials gain weight – especially if they are on a high starting dose and if they were underweight pre-treatment. Reported evidence to date suggests that olanzapine is relatively less likely to produce sexual dysfunction. In general weight gain and sexual dysfunction are of great concern to people taking antipsychotics and the side-effect profile of any antipsychotic may affect compliance. Olanzapine's general efficacy and side-effect profile suggest an important role in the first line management of psychotic disorders.

Introduction

Olanzapine* demonstrates mesolimbic selectivity, blocks conditioned avoidance at lower doses than those inducing catalepsy, substitutes for clozapine in a drug discrimination assay, produces a modest rise in prolactin, produces few extrapyramidal side-effects and reduces positive and negative symptoms of schizophrenia in a similar way to clozapine[20]. However, despite this 'atypical' profile olanzapine has a weaker alpha-2 blockade than clozapine or risperidone. It has relatively high affinity for muscarinic, 5-HT_2, and D_1, D_2 and D_4 receptors. Studies indicate a good response in patients with schizophrenia with few extrapyramidal side-effects (EPSEs). Administration is currently via the oral route. Coated tablets exist in 2.5 mg, 5 mg, 7.5 mg or 10 mg doses. A rapidly dissolving tablet (Zyprexa Velotab) has recently been made available in 5 mg and 10 mg doses. An intramuscular form has been researched for use in agitation[42].

Clinical indications

The licensed indication is for schizophrenia and related psychoses. The following additional indications are derived from MEDLINE and PSY-CLIT database searches and are not necessarily endorsed by the manufacturer. The primary indications for olanzapine appear to be

---

*2-methyl-4-(4-methyl-1-piperazinyl)-10H-thieno[2,3-b][1,5] benzodiazepine.

undoubtedly adult schizophrenia and related psychoses[4]. Adolescent schizophrenia[15], affective symptoms in schizophrenia[37], schizoaffective disorder[36], bipolar affective disorder and mania[14,24,43], affective psychoses[9,41], behaviour and symptom control in dementia are secondary indications. The relatively greater ability to reduce negative symptoms compared to conventional antipsychotics and risperidone provides an additional indication[35,39].

Olanzapine and other antipsychotics have been proposed as first-line treatments for schizophrenia and there is some rationale for this[17]. Clozapine has not been generally used as a first-line treatment due to its potential for agranulocytosis. Compared to conventional antipsychotics such as chlorpromazine and haloperidol, olanzapine and other second generation antipsychotics tend to provide superior efficacy, fewer side-effects, and thus the possibility of better patient compliance. The best use of drugs such as olanzapine may be in patients at the beginning of their illness as a first-line treatment of schizophrenia and in patients who require switching from conventional antipsychotics because of difficulties with side-effects or treatment-resistant symptoms.

Health economic studies are few at this time. There is hope that, although the direct costs of olanzapine are high, indirect benefits including reduced needs for hospitalisation, better quality of life[13] and improved patient compliance may provide economic arguments for use over apparently cheaper, traditional antipsychotics.

Almond and O'Donnell[2] performed a cost analysis of the treatment of schizophrenia in the UK. They quote the annual direct and indirect costs of schizophrenia in the UK in the 1990s to be £2.6 billion. They concluded that, compared to haloperidol, olanzapine generated savings by reducing use of medical services. These savings offset the higher prescriptions costs to produce an approximately cost-neutral comparison. Taking everything into consideration, on average haloperidol appeared to be some £160 per annum more costly than olanzapine. Glazer and Johnstone[12] performed a randomised, double-blind study comparing the use of medical services and the cost of treatment for 817 people with schizophrenia treated with olanzapine or haloperidol. Looking at comprehensive health care costs including the costs of study medications, the total cost of health care for olanzapine-treated patients was reduced by an average of $431 per month in comparison with haloperidol-treated patients during the first 6 weeks of treatment. Over the year, the total cost of care among olanzapine responders was reduced by an average of $345 per month in comparison with haloperidol responders.

There is evidence for the use of olanzapine in treatment-resistant schizophrenia[19], and in conventional antipsychotic-induced tardive dyskinesia[18,22], suggesting some indications for switching therapy from existing antipsychotics where problems exist.

Initial research on second-generation antipsychotics has tended to focus on younger adults, but studies using older patients are emerging. Street et al.[30] from Lilly's own research laboratories have published the results of a double-blind, randomised, placebo-controlled trial of olanzapine used for psychotic and behavioural symptoms in Alzheimer Disease patients. Low-dose olanzapine (5–10 mg/day) produced significant improvements in 206 nursing home residents compared to placebo.

There is a suggestion in current research that olanzapine may be useful in Tourette's syndrome[28], although double-blind randomised trails are awaited. Fourteen patients with a mean age of 32.6 years were enrolled in this study and improvements found on the Yale Global Tic Severity Scale (YGTSS), Fischer Symptom Check List–Neuroleptika and the Clinical Global Impression Severity Scale (CGI). Seven patients had not responded to, or not tolerated, other antipsychotics and seven were neuroleptic-naïve.

Clinical efficacy

In Eli Lilly's clinical trials by Tran, Tollefson and others 335 patients with schizophrenia were randomised to five treatment groups:
- placebo;
- olanzapine low-dose range (2.5–7.5 mg);
- olanzapine medium-dose range (7.5–12.5 mg);
- olanzapine high-dose range (12.5–17.5 mg);
- haloperidol (10–20 mg).

The trial lasted 6 weeks and involved weekly

evaluations. Patients receiving olanzapine had few EPSEs, with no dystonic reactions – contrasted with 13% of the haloperidol group, although other pre-marketing trials did have some reports of dystonia. It was the high-dose treatment group that produced BPRS rating reductions numerically superior to haloperidol and statistically significant compared to placebo. SANS score comparison showed a similar statistically better reduction for the high-dose olanzapine group compared to haloperidol and placebo.

152 patients were involved in a double-blind multicentre six-week study where the 10 mg olanzapine dosage was well tolerated and produced a significant effect against positive and negative symptoms compared to placebo[4]. Scales used included the Brief Psychiatric Rating Scale (BPRS), Positive and Negative Symptom Scale (PANSS) and Clinical Global Impression – severity of illness (CGI). Tollefson et al.[36] performed a multicentre, double-blind trial of 1,996 patients which showed that olanzapine was superior to haloperidol at reducing overall BPRS and negative symptoms. A reduction in affective symptoms was also noted compared to haloperidol.

Negative symptoms are sometimes attributed to permanent frontal lobe deficits, and therefore sometimes deemed irreversible. Tollefson and Sanger's study of negative symptoms[35] looked at 335 patients comparing haloperidol and olanzapine over 52 weeks. A path analysis was used to determine to what extent the treatment on treatment symptoms was direct or indirect. Compared to haloperidol or placebo, olanzapine was significantly more likely to directly improve Schedule for the Assessment of Negative Symptoms (SANS) scores, particularly with regard to affective blunting and apathy.

Maintenance therapy with olanzapine promises fewer relapses than with conventional agents such as haloperidol. In a study by Tran et al.[40] the estimated one-year relapse rate with oral olanzapine was 19% whereas oral haloperidol's estimated relapse rate was 28%.

Side-effects

Compared with traditional antipsychotics olanzapine has a vastly improved side-effect profile[6]. The reduced potential for inducing extrapyramidal side-effects[38], tardive dyskinesia[34] and improving quality of life provide a rationale for the early use of this agent.

Although only licensed up to 20 mg a day, higher doses are sometimes used in resistant schizophrenia (for example, 30 mg olanzapine daily). Higher doses such as these may be associated with increased reports of side-effects including acute extrapyramidal side-effects – akathisia and parkinsonism – although symptoms were reported as mild. Mild daytime drowsiness and dry mouth also occurred[27].

The most common side-effects appear to be somnolence and weight gain. About 40% of patients gain weight – especially if on a high starting dose and if they were underweight pretreatment.

Sexual dysfunction is a problem for many patients, although sexual dysfunction in schizophrenia does not appear to be primarily attributable to drugs. Untreated patients with schizophrenia have more sexual problems than controls[1].

Results from Eli Lilly's clinical trials of olanzapine have yielded the data shown in Table 9.2.

Recent work by Tollefson et al.[33] from an international multicentre, double-blind parallel trial looks at olanzapine versus haloperidol in first-episode psychosis. Olanzapine was significantly better than haloperidol in reducing average BPRS total scores, BPRS negative scores, PANSS total scores and PANSS positive scores. Haloperidol-prescribed patients had significantly more EPS.

The weight gain produced by olanzapine has been studied more over recent years. Taylor and McAskill[32] rated olanzapine's potential to produce weight gain as second only to that of clozapine. The weight gain appears to be linked to a rise in serum triglycerides, much as clozapine seems to do. Osser et al.'s study[23] of 25 inpatients treated with olanzapine revealed that, after 12 weeks on a mean dose of about 14 mg/day, weight increased a mean of 5.4 kg whilst fasting triglycerides increased by a mean of 60 mg/dL. Of further concern was the fact that the triglyceride increase was even larger when the investigators excluded 8 patients who received various interventions to lower lipid levels (for example, pravastatin, low-fat diet). There appeared to be a strong association between weight gain and triglyceride change.

There has been interest in the effects of olanzapine and clozapine on the insulin regulatory system and an associated induction of diabetes.

Table 9.1:

Side-effect	Olanzapine (n=1796)	Haloperidol (n=810)
Postural hypotension	2%	1%
Constipation	5%	4%
Dry mouth	7%	4%
Somnolence	16%	15%
Hostility	6%	5%
Headache	11%	13%
Diarrhoea	3%	3%
Akathisia	6%	21%
Confusion	1%	2%
Dyskinesia	0%	2%
Tremor	3%	13%
Anxiety	6%	8%
Agitation	8%	9%
Rash	2%	1%

Table 9.2:

Event	Number of reports. Total $N=2,500$	Percentage reporting
Decreased libido	23	0.9%
Increased libido	18	0.7%
Impotence	11	0.7%
Abnormal ejaculation	3	0.2%
Priapism	1	0.1% (Denominator = only males)
Anorgasmia	1	0.0%

Liebzeit, Markowitz and Caley[16] looked at 35 cases of induced or exacerbated diabetes in the published literature. Of these, the vast majority of cases implicate clozapine ($n = 20$) and olanzapine ($n = 15$). Diabetic ketoacidosis was often the presenting symptom.

Olanzapine has been linked with a clinically important and significant risk of diabetes in a population-based case-control study[44].

There has been a published report of two cases of reversible neutropenia associated with olanzapine[29]. The neutropenia was noted 17 days after the first exposure to olanzapine in one case and more than 5 months after first exposure to olanzapine in the second case.

The unwanted similarities to clozapine may also extend to abnormalities on EEGs. Clozapine is known to reduce the overall epileptic threshold and can induce epileptic seizures. In a very small series of nine patients on olanzapine and nine on clozapine, Schuld et al.[26] found that olanzapine induced significant EEG slowing, but less frequently (in 4 of the patients) and less pronounced than in the patients on clozapine. Olanzapine had no significant effect an epileptiform activity, but in one patient, an isolated sharp/slow-wave complex was observed. The authors qualify their work, stating that no case of seizure induction has been reported so far with olanzapine. Personal observations of patients in my own clinic have seen patients discontinuing use of the drug after isolated olfactory hallucinations related to starting the drug and isolated somnambulism. Both symptoms discontinued after the patients stopped the drug. Schuld et al.[26] point out that this aspect of olanzapine deserves further attention.

Drug interactions

Olanzapine generally shows a low potential for drug interactions. The metabolism of olanzapine includes N-glucuronidation. This lowers its overall sensitivity to drugs that might induce or inhibit its own metabolism via CYP or flavin-containing monooxygenase (FMO) systems[10]. In *in-vitro* studies olanzapine's percentage inhibition of P450 cytochromes has been shown to be < 0.3%, suggesting a low potential for interaction with compounds metabolised by these enzymes[25].

Carbamazepine, by induction, increases clearance of olanzapine by up to 44%. Smoking also induces the metabolism of olanzapine.

Olanzapine is 93% protein-bound and so there is a potential for displacing other drugs from plasma proteins.

Comparisons with other novel antipsychotics

In terms of binding with rat and human tissue receptors, olanzapine had high affinity for dopamine D_1, D_2, D_4, serotonin $5HT_{2A}$, $5HT_{2C}$, $5HT_3$, $alpha_1$-adrenergic, histamine H_1, and five muscarinic receptor subtypes. Olanzapine has a lower affinity for $alpha_2$-adrenergic receptors and a relatively low affinity for $5HT_1$ subtypes, GABAA, beta-adrenergic receptors, and benzodiazepine binding sites[21]. The binding profile of olanzapine is probably therefore closer to that of clozapine than other antipsychotics such as haloperidol, risperidone, remoxipride, and quetiapine[5].

The hope of many clinicians was for an atypical antipsychotic, effective in conventional treatment-resistant patients, but without the haematological side-effects of clozapine. Although there is some evidence for an effect in about a third of treatment-resistant patients[19], the effect does not appear to be as marked as with clozapine, and the indications for clozapine appear unchanged by the introduction of olanzapine[11].

Following switching to olanzapine from an older antipsychotic there may be an increase in fertility and physicians should be aware of a need for patient counselling and possibly changes in contraceptive use[7].

Compared to risperidone olanzapine is less likely to induce extrapyramidal side-effects, hyperprolactinemia, and sexual dysfunction[38]. Although both risperidone and olanzapine appear equally effective in the treatment of positive symptoms, results of the Tran study indicated that olanzapine had significantly greater efficacy in reducing negative symptoms.

Compared to risperidone olanzapine appears to have the following features:

- greater tolerability;
- better at reducing affective symptoms;
- possibly better at improving patient quality of life and interpersonal relationships;
- statistically better improvements in PANSS scores and fewer relapses;
- fewer EPS and less sexual dysfunction;
- less likely to elevate prolactin levels.

Olanzapine and risperidone are two of the novel or second-generation antipsychotics, but they differ in terms of chemical structures, overall receptor-binding affinity, animal neuropharmacology, pharmacokinetics and risk/benefit profiles. An international, randomised double-blind parallel study has been performed comparing risperidone and olanzapine in DSM-IV schizophrenia, schizophreniform disorder and schizoaffective disorder. The study involved an 8-week acute phase followed by a 20-week extension phase. The dose ranges for olanzapine were 5–20 mg/day, and 4–12 mg/day for risperidone. Statistically significantly, more olanzapine-treated patients completed the 28 weeks than risperidone-treated patients (68% versus 48%, $p = .028$). Both risperidone and olanzapine appeared to be effective antipsychotics for positive and negative symptomatology. Olanzapine demonstrated superiority over risperidone in reducing mood symptoms, providing high clinical response rates, maintaining response and improving interpersonal relationships.

After 28 weeks of therapy olanzapine showed statistically better improvements in PANSS scores and fewer relapses than risperidone. At 6 months the rates of relapse were 11% for olanzapine and 29% for risperidone. Olanzapine patients have statistically fewer EPS and sexual dysfunction, measured by subjective and objective rating scales. Olanzapine patients were less likely to have elevated prolactin levels than the risperidone group.

Conclusions

Olanzapine is a second-generation antipsychotic launched in the UK in October 1996. The clinical impression is of a useful antipsychotic with few EPSEs and with a potential to reduce positive and negative symptoms to a better degree than some conventional antipsychotics. There is good tolerability, but a major problem with the drug appears to be weight gain, associated with a rise in triglycerides. About 40% of patients gain weight – especially if they are on a high starting dose and if they were underweight pre-treatment. Since its launch the drug has become widely used and as might be predicted some revision has taken place amongst its prescribers in terms of their perception of the drug[3].

Olanzapine's general efficacy and side-effect profile suggest that olanzapine should have a role in the initial management of psychotic disorders.

References

1. Aizenberg D, Zemishlany Z, Dorfman-Etrog P, Weizman A (1995). Sexual dysfunction in male schizophrenic patients. *J. Clin. Psychiatry,* 56(4): 137–141.
2. Almond S, O'Donnell O (1998). Cost analysis of the treatment of schizophrenia in the UK. A comparison of olanzapine and haloperidol. *Pharmacoeconomics,*13,(SPt2),575–588.
3. Anonymous (2000). Olanzapine. Keep an eye on this neuroleptic [see comments]. Comment in: *Can Fam Physician* (2000 May) 46:1022; Comment in: *Can Fam Physician* (2000 Aug) 46:1565–6, 1569. *Canadian Family Physician,* 46:322–6,330–6,2000Feb.
4. Beasley CM, Tollefson G, Tran P, Satterlee W, Sanger T, Hamilton S (1996). Olanzapine versus placebo and haloperidol: acute phase results of the North American double-blind olanzapine trial. *Neuropsychopharmacology,* 14(2):111– 23.
5. Bymaster FP, Calligaro DO, Falcone JF, Marsh RD, Moore NA, Tye NC, Seeman P, Wong DT (1996). Radioreceptor binding profile of the atypical antipsychotic olanzapine. *Neuropsychopharmacology,*14(2):87–96.
6. Casey DE (1996). Side effect profiles of new antipsychotic agents. *J. Clin. Psychiatry,* 57(Suppl 11):40–5;discussion46–52.
7. Currier GW, Simpson GM (1998). Antipsychotic medications and fertility. *Psychiatric-Services,*vol.49(2):175–6.
8. Czekalla J, Beasley CM Jr, Dellva MA, Berg PH, Grundy S (2001). Analysis of the QTc interval during olanzapine treatment of patients with schizophrenia and related psychosis. *Journal of Clinical Psychiatry,* 62(3):191–8,2001Mar.
9. Debattista C, Solvason HB, Belanoff J, Schatzberg AF (1997). Treatment of psychotic depression. [letter] *Am. J. Psychiatry,* 154(11): 1625–6.
10. Ereshefsky L (1996). Pharmacokinetics and drug interactions: update for new antipsychotics. *J. Clin. Psychiatry,*57(Suppl11):12–25.
11. Ganguli R, Brar JS (1998). The effects of risperidone and olanzapine on the indications for clozapine. *Psychopharmacol. Bull.,34(1):83–7.*
12. Glazer WM, Johnstone BM (1997). Pharmacoeconomic evaluation of antipsychotic therapy for schizophrenia. *J. Clin. Psychiatry,* 58(Suppl 10):50–4.
13. Hamilton SH, Revicki DA, Genduso LA, Beasley CM (1998). Olanzapine versus placebo and haloperidol: quality of life and efficacy results of the North American double-blind trial. *Neuropsychopharmacology,*18(1):41–9.
14. Ketter TA, Winsberg ME, DeGolia SG, *et al.* (1998). Rapid efficacy of olanzapine augmentation in nonpsychotic bipolar mixed states. *J. Clin. Psychiatry,*59(2):83–5.
15. Kumra S, Jacobsen LK, Lenane M, *et al.* (1998). Childhood-onset schizophrenia: an open-label study of olanzapine in adolescents. *J. Am. Acad. Child.Adolesc.Psychiatry,* 37(4): 377–85.
16. Liebzeit KA, Markowitz JS, Caley CF (2001). New onset diabetes and atypical antipsychotics. *European Neuropsychopharmacology,* 11(1):25–32,2001Feb.
17. Lieberman JA (1996). Atypical antipsychotic drugs as a first-line treatment of schizophrenia: a rationale and hypothesis. *J. Clin. Psychiatry,* 57(Suppl11):68–71.
18. Littrell KH, Johnson CG, Littrell S, Peabody CD (1998). Marked reduction of tardive dyskinesia with olanzapine. *Archives-of-General-Psychiatry,* vol.55(3):279–280.
19. Martin J, Gomez JC, Garcia-Bernardo E, *et al.* (1997). Olanzapine in treatment-refractory schizophrenia: results of an open-label study. The Spanish Group for the Study of Olanzapine in Treatment-Refractory Schizophrenia. *J. Clin. Psychiatry,* 58(11): 479–83.
20. Moore NA (1995). Letter to the Editor. *J. Psychopharmacology,*9,155.
21. Nutt DJ (1994). Putting the 'A' in atypical: does alpha-2 adrenoceptor antagonism account for the therapeutic advantage of new antipsychotics? *J. Psychopharmacol.,*8,193–5.
22. O'Brien J, Barber R (1998). Marked improvement in tardive dyskinesia following treatment with olanzapine in an elderly subject. *Br. J. Psychiatry,*172:186.
23. Osser DN, Najarian DM, Dufresne RL (1999). Olanzapine increases weight and serum triglyceride levels. *Journal of Clinical Psychiatry,* 60(11): 767–70,1999Nov.
24. Ravindran AV, Jones BW, al-Zaid K, Lapierre YD (1997). Effective treatment of mania with olanzapine: 2 case reports. *J. Psychiatry. Neurosci.,*22(5):345–6.

25. Ring BJ, Binkley SN, Vandenbranden M, Wrighton SA (1996). In vitro interaction of the antipsychotic agent olanzapine with human cytochromes P450 CYP2C9, CYP2C19, CYP2D6 and CYP3A. *Br. J. Clin.Pharmacol.*, 41(3):181–6.
26. Schuld A, Kuhn M, Haack M, Kraus T, HinzeSelch D, Lechner C, Pollmacher T (2000). A comparison of the effects of clozapine and olanzapine on the EEG in patients with schizophrenia. *Pharmacopsychiatry,* 33(3):109–11, 2000 May.
27. Sheitman BB, Lindgren JC, Early J, Sved M (1997). High-dose olanzapine for treatment-resistant schizophrenia. *American Journal of Psychiatry*,vol.154(11):1626.
28. Stamenkovic M, Schindler SD, Aschauer HN, De Zwaan M, Willinger U, Resinger E, Kasper S (2000). Effective open-label treatment of Tourette's disorder with olanzapine. *International Clinical Psychopharmacology,* 15(1):23–8.
29. Steinwachs A, Grohmann R, Pedrosa F, Ruther E, Schwerdtner I (1999). Two cases of olanzapine-induced reversible neutropenia. *Pharmacopsychiatry,*32(4):154–6.
30. Street JS, Clark WS, Gannon KS, Cummings JL, Bymaster FP, Tamura RN, Mitan SJ, Kadam DL, Sanger TM, Feldman PD, Tollefson GD, Breier A (2000). Olanzapine treatment of psychotic and behavioral symptoms in patients with Alzheimer disease in nursing care facilities: a double-blind, randomized, placebo-controlled trial. The HGEU Study Group. *Archives of General Psychiatry,* 57(10): 968–76.
31. Stockton ME, Rasmussen K (1996). Electrophysiological effects of olanzapine, a novel atypical antipsychotic, on A9 and A10 dopamine neurons. *Neuropsychopharmacology,* 14:97–104.
32. Taylor DM, McAskill R (2000). Atypical antipsychotics and weight gain – a systematic review. *Acta Psychiatrica Scandinavica,* 101(6): 416–32.
33. Tollefson GD, Sanger TM, Lieberman JA (1997). Olanzapine versus haloperidol in the treatment of first episode psychosis. *Schizophrenia Research,* 24Nos.1–2.
34. Tollefson GD, Beasley CM, Tamura RN, Tran PV, Potvin JH (1997). Blind, controlled, long-term study of the comparative incidence of treatment-emergent tardive dyskinesia with olanzapine or haloperidol. *Am. J. Psychiatry,* 154(9):1248–54.
35. Tollefson GD, Sanger TM (1997). Negative symptoms: a path analytic approach to a double-blind, placebo- and haloperidol-controlled clinical trial with olanzapine. *Am. J. Psychiatry,* 154(4):466–74.
36. Tollefson GD, Beasley CM, Tran PV, Street JS, Krueger JA, Tamura RN, Graffeo KA, Thieme ME (1997). Olanzapine versus haloperidol in the treatment of schizophrenia and schizoaffective and schizophreniform disorders: results of an international collaborative trial. *Am. J. Psychiatry,*154(4):457–65.
37. Tollefson GD, Sanger TM, Lu Y, Thieme ME (1998). Depressive signs and symptoms in schizophrenia: a prospective blinded trial of olanzapine and haloperidol. *Arch. Gen. Psychiatry,*55(3):250–8.
38. Tran PV, Dellva MA, Tollefson GD, Beasley CM, Potvin JH, Kiesler GM (1997). Extrapyramidal symptoms and tolerability of olanzapine versus haloperidol in the acute treatment of schizophrenia. *J. Clin. Psychiatry,*58(5):205–11.
39. Tran PV, Hamilton SH, Kuntz AJ, Potvin JH, Andersen SW, Beasley C, Tollefson GD (1997). Double-blind comparison of olanzapine versus risperidone in the treatment of schizophrenia and other psychotic disorders. *J. Clin. Psychopharmacol.,*17(5):407–18.
40. Tran PV, Dellva MA, Tollefson GD, Wentley AL, Beasley CM (1998). Oral olanzapine versus oral haloperidol in the maintenance treatment of schizophrenia and related psychoses. *B. J. Psychiatry,*172,499–505.
41. Weisler RH, Ahearn EP, Davidson JR, Wallace CD (1997). Adjunctive use of olanzapine in mood disorders: five case reports. *Ann. Clin. Psychiatry,*259–62.
42. Wright P, Birkett M, David SR, Meehan K, FerchlandI,AlakaKJ,SaundersJC,KruegerJ,Bradley P, San L, Bernardo M, Reinstein M, Breier A (2001). Double-blind, placebo-controlled comparison of intramuscular olanzapine and intramuscular haloperidol in the treatment of acute agitation in schizophrenia. *American Journal of Psychiatry,*158(7):1149–51,2001Jul.
43. Zarate CA, Narendran R, Tohen M, Greaney JJ, Berman A, Pike S, Madrid A (1998). Clinical predictors of acute response with olanzapine in psychotic mood disorders. *J. Clin. Psychiatry,* 59(1):24–8.
44. Koro CE, Fedder DO, L'Italien GJ, Weiss SS, Magder LS, Kreyenbuhl J, Revicki DA, Buchanan RW (2002). Assessment of independent effet of olanzapine and risperidone on risk of diabetes among patients with schizophrenia: population based nested case-control study. *BMJ,*325:243–5.

Chapter 10
Focus on Quetiapine

Dr Ben Green

Summary

Quetiapine fumarate is a novel dibenzothiazepine antipsychotic developed by AstraZeneca and marketed under the trade name 'Seroquel'. Quetiapine is well tolerated and clinically effective in the treatment of schizophrenia.

The initial hope of investigators was that quetiapine would have antipsychotic potential and that it might share some of the properties of clozapine without its toxicity to white blood cells. The effective dosage range is usually 300–450 mg/day split into two doses. The dose is titrated upwards from 25 mg twice daily from day 1 to 300 mg/day on day 4. Elderly patients or patients with liver problems should be started on lower doses. It is both superior to placebo and comparable to haloperidol in reducing positive symptoms at doses ranging from 150 mg/day to 750 mg/day, and is an effective treatment for negative symptoms.

Somnolence is the most common adverse event. Abnormalities of the QT interval on ECG appear very infrequently and there is no need for a baseline ECG or blood pressure monitoring, as used to be the case with sertindole. There is no need for haematological monitoring as with clozapine. Quetiapine, across the full dosage range, is associated with no greater extrapyramidal symptoms than placebo, indeed it may even reverse previous EPS and improve tardive dyskinesia. Quetiapine has a favourable weight profile.

Quetiapine appears to be less likely to induce sexual dysfunction than olanzapine, haloperidol or risperidone.

Quetiapine has equal efficacy to risperidone in the treatment of schizophrenia, but produces fewer extrapyramidal side-effects.

Quetiapine's general efficacy and side-effect profile suggest that it deserves a major place in the initial and long-term management of schizophrenia and associated disorders.

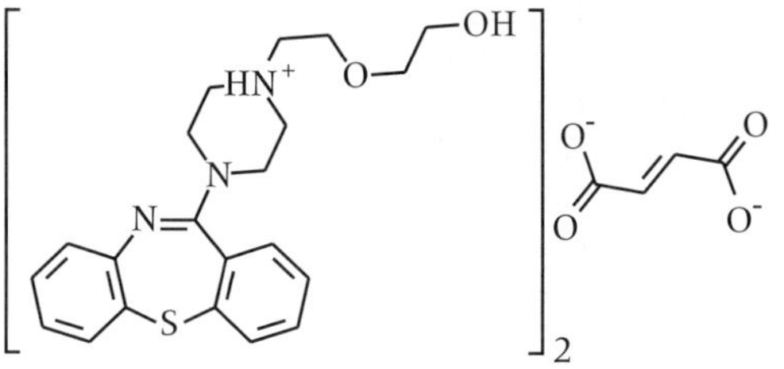

Figure 10.1: The molecular structure of quetiapine.

Introduction

Quetiapine fumarate* is a novel dibenzothiazepine antipsychotic developed by Zeneca Pharmaceuticals. It is marketed under the trade name 'Seroquel'. Quetiapine is well tolerated and clinically effective in the treatment of schizophrenia.

Dosage regime

The usual effective dosage range for the treatment of manic episodes associated with bipolar disorder is in the range of 400–800 mg. The total daily dose for the first four days of therapy is 100 mg (day 1), 200 mg (day 2), 300 mg (day 3) and 400 mg (day 4). Further adjustments up to 800 mg per day by day 6 should be in increments of no greater than 200 mg per day.

Clinical indications

Licensed indications vary from country to country. The following indications are derived from MEDLINE, Cochrane and PSYCLIT database searches. The primary indications are adult schizophrenia and manic episodes associated with bipolar disorder. Additional studies may support quetiapine's use in: affective and aggressive symptoms in schizophrenia[9], adolescent schizophrenia, schizoaffective disorder, bipolar affective disorder and mania, affective psychoses, and behaviour and symptom control in dementia

---

*Bis [2-(2-[4-(dibenzo[b,f][1,4]thiazepin-11-yl]ethoxy)ethanol] fumarate (IUPAC) (ICI 204,636)

could form secondary indications, but more studies are awaited.

Quetiapine and other antipsychotics have been proposed as first-line treatments for schizophrenia and there is some rationale for this[15]. Clozapine has not generally been used as a first-line treatment owing to its potential for agranulocytosis. Compared to conventional antipsychotics such as chlorpromazine and haloperidol, quetiapine and other atypical antipsychotics provide superior efficacy or fewer side-effects, particularly extrapyramidal symptoms (EPS), and the possibility of better patient compliance. Drugs such as quetiapine may therefore be particularly appropriate in patients at the beginning of their illness as a first-line treatment of schizophrenia.

Some abnormal involuntary movement disorders such as tardive dyskinesia may improve with quetiapine (after previous treatment with conventional antipsychotics), as dopamine D_2 receptor occupancy reduces[25].

Some evidence exists that psychotic patients with diagnoses of bipolar disorder, manic, mixed, or depressed and schizoaffective disorder, bipolar type have been found to respond well to quetiapine[27].

Pre-clinical studies

In rodents, quetiapine produced mild levels of catalepsy, which suggested antipsychotic potential. It has a low propensity to cause dystonia in drug-naïve or haloperidol-sensitised monkeys[10]. Rats treated with apomorphine (APO) exhibit deficits in prepulse inhibition (PPI) of the acoustic startle response. This is thought to model schizophrenia. Clozapine restores PPI in APO-treated rats and this ability tends to correlate ($RS = 0.991$) with the clinical potency of antipsychotics. Quetiapine similarly restores deficits in PPI[23].

In vitro binding affinity is more for 5-HT_2 receptors than dopamine DA_2 receptors and *in vivo* dopamine DA_2- and 5-HT_2-receptor occupancies are 27% and 58%, respectively (see Table 10.1). Conventional antipsychotics block up to 80% of DA_2 receptors as measured using positron emission tomography scans – see Figure 10.2[13]. Clozapine and quetiapine occupy about 30%, which may explain their low propensity to cause EPS. Only clozapine and quetiapine share a low affinity for dopamine

Table 10.1: Receptor affinities in the brain.

Receptor	Quetiapine (IC50, nM)	Clozapine (IC50, nM)
DA_2	329	132
DA_1	1268	322
5-HT_2	148	20
5-HT_{1A}	717	316
alpha$_1$	94	50
alpha$_2$	271	28
H_1	30	23
sigma	90	>10 000
Muscarinic	>10 000	287
Benzodiazepine	>5000	>5000

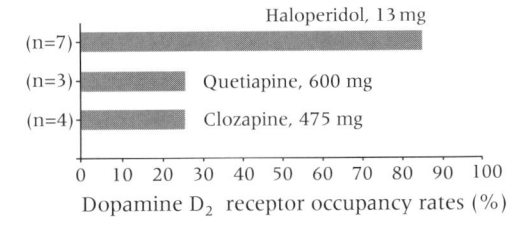

Figure 10.2: Positron emission tomography (PET) derived DA_2 occupancy comparing quetiapine, clozapine and haloperidol (after Kasper[13]).

DA_2 receptors and an antagonistic action at alpha$_2$ adrenoceptors[20]. The clinical import of this is not yet clear.

Compared with clozapine, quetiapine has much the same ratio of DA_2/5-HT_2 occupancy[6].

Quetiapine binds to dopamine DA_2 receptors in the striatum and occupies 44% of receptors 2 hours (t_{max}) after the last dose. After 26 hours, occupancy dropped to the same level as in untreated healthy volunteers. Serotonin 5-HT_2 receptor blockade in the frontal cortex was 72% after 2 hours, which fell to 50% after 26 hours. The terminal plasma half-life of quetiapine was found to be 5.3 hours[6].

In a PET study by Kapur *et al.*[12] quetiapine showed a transiently high D_2 occupancy, which decreased to very low levels by the end of the dosing interval. The drug's low D_2 occupancy could explain its freedom from extrapyramidal symptoms and prolactin level elevation. The data suggest that transient D_2 occupancy may be sufficient for its antipsychotic effect.

Pharmacokinetics and metabolism

Quetiapine is rapidly absorbed and has linear pharmacokinetics. The mean half-life for 375 mg/day is 6.9 h. The steady-state pharmacokinetics appear to be the same for men and women. At 2, 12 and 24 h post-dose, quetiapine's 5-HT$_2$ occupancy was 72%, 48% and 50%, respectively. It is only moderately bound to plasma protein (83%). Quetiapine is extensively metabolised by the liver involving mainly sulphoxidation by cytochrome P450 3A4[8]. It is extensively metabolised to over 20 metabolites – some are active, but the concentration of these active metabolites is low compared with the parent compound. Quetiapine is eliminated primarily in the form of metabolites, only 5% being excreted unchanged. About 73% is excreted in the urine and 21% in the faeces.

Oral clearance in the elderly is half that of younger patients. Clearance is also reduced by hepatic or renal impairment.

Clinical efficacy

In one of Zeneca's initial clinical trials, five fixed doses of quetiapine were studied to investigate the dose–response relationship[1]. Outcome measures included the Brief Psychiatric Rating Scale (BPRS), Clinical Global Impression (CGI) and the Modified Scale for the Assessment of Negative Symptoms (SANS). 361 patients with acute exacerbations of chronic schizophrenia (DSM-III-R) from 26 US centres entered this double-blind, placebo-controlled trial. After a single-blind, placebo-washout phase, patients were randomised to double-blind treatment with quetiapine (75, 150, 300, 600 or 750 mg daily), haloperidol (12 mg daily), or placebo, and evaluated weekly for 6 weeks. At the end of the study, significant differences ($p < 0.05$, analysis of covariance) were identified between the four highest doses of quetiapine and placebo for BPRS total, BPRS positive-symptom cluster and CGI Severity of Illness item scores, and between quetiapine 300 mg and placebo for SANS summary score. The study's scales did not show a statistically significant difference between quetiapine and haloperidol. No significant safety problems manifested as the dose increased. Quetiapine at any of the doses seemed no different from placebo in terms of the incidences of extrapyramidal symptoms.

Similar efficacy studies demonstrate that quetiapine is as effective as chlorpromazine[1,3,17,21]. A 6-week, double-blind, randomised, multicentre, parallel-group study compared the efficacy of quetiapine (n = 101) with that of chlorpromazine (n = 100) in hospital patients with acute exacerbation schizophrenia or schizophreniform disorder. The mean daily doses of quetiapine and chlorpromazine at the end of the study were 407 mg and 384 mg, respectively. Both treatments reduced positive and negative symptoms, with a trend towards superior efficacy for quetiapine. The quetiapine group had lower incidences of adverse events and lower incidences of extra-pyramidal symptoms requiring treatment with anti-cholinergics. Quetiapine was not associated with an increase in serum prolactin, supporting the preclinical profile of quetiapine as an atypical antipsychotic agent.

There are now several short-term (6 weeks or so) double-blind randomised clinical trials on quetiapine's efficacy, producing data from over a thousand patients (referred to above). Quetiapine showed consistent efficacy in the treatment of positive symptoms using the Brief Psychiatric Rating Scale (BPRS) positive symptom cluster. Longer-term efficacy studies are being performed which may demonstrate quetiepine improves mood in patients with schizophrenia according to ratings on the BPRS item scores for depressive mood, anxiety, guilt and tension.

Srisurapanont et al.[22] published a typically cautious Cochrane review which concluded that quetiapine had a slightly superior efficacy to haloperidol, but a similar efficacy to chlorpromazine.

Copolov et al.[5] performed a six-week multicentre, double-blind, randomised, parallel-group trial comparing quetiapine with haloperidol (455 mg and 8 mg mean total daily doses, respectively) in 448 in-patients with schizophrenia. They found that quetiapine had a comparable efficacy to haloperidol and lacked haloperidol's adverse effects on prolactin and EPS.

There is less data about the elderly than there is about younger adults. Seven elderly hospital in-patients between 61 and 72 years of age had schizophrenia, schizoaffective disorder, or bipolar disorder were treated by Madhusoodanan et al.[16]. All seven had been treated before with conventional antipsychotics or other atypical antipsychotics. Four patients responded to treatment; three did not respond. Pre-existing extrapyramidal symptoms (EPS) diminished in three patients. Hypotension, dizziness and somnolence occurred in two patients. Overall the authors concluded that quetiapine was a safe and effective medication for the elderly.

Besides its overall antipsychotic effects on traditional psychotic symptoms, improvement has been noted compared with haloperidol in neuropsychological functioning, specifically: verbal reasoning and fluency skills and immediate recall, with additional improvements on executive skills and visuomotor tracking[19].

According to data from the QUEST trial[24,] quetiapine is as effective as risperidone in treating schizophrenia, but produces significantly fewer extrapyramidal side-effects than risperidone (odds ratio 0.39, $p = 0.0326$).

Side-effects

Several thousand patients have now received quetiapine over varying treatment course lengths culminating in several thousand patient years of exposure to the drug. Somnolence is the most common side-effect leading to withdrawal from treatment in 1.4% of patients.

Interestingly, placebo-controlled studies of quetiapine identified no significant difference between quetiapine and placebo for dystonia, akathisia and Parkinsonism[21]. There appear to be no dose-related increases in the incidences of EPS with quetiapine, unlike some other antipsychotics – such as risperidone. Only 8.6% of patients in clinical trials required anticholinergic medication compared with 12.6% of patients on placebo. There were significantly lower incidences of EPS in comparisons of quetiapine and haloperidol.

Patient satisfaction is rarely measured in clinical trials, but it is probably a crucial factor in compliance. A total of 76% of 129 patients on quetiapine for at least six months in an open-label study extension reported that they were very or extremely satisfied with their treatment in a questionnaire-based study for AstraZeneca[14]. 74% of these long-term patients reported no side-effects and 23% only mild side-effects, in the previous month of therapy; 97% said they preferred quetiapine to previous medications.

Quetiapine is generally well tolerated by the elderly, although lower doses need to be given

Table 10.2: Incidence of side-effects with quetiapine.

Adverse event	Percentage of patients in Phase II/III studies ($n = 1710$)
Somnolence	18.2
Dizziness	7.5
Asthenia	4.3
Postural hypotension	5.8
Tachycardia	4.2
Constipation	5.5
Dry mouth	7.1
Dyspepsia	3.4
Sexual dysfunction	0.5

because of its pharmacokinetics. There are negligible EPSs in the elderly. Somnolence, dizziness and postural hypotension are the most frequent side-effects in the elderly[26].

Reproductive and hormonal adverse events (such as gynaecomastia, amenorrhoea, abnormal ejaculation, lactation) occur very rarely, probably since prolactin levels are no different from placebo across the dose range[7].

There is relatively little experience of the drug in overdose. Pollak and Zbuk[18] report that quetiapine is safer than conventional antipsychotic agents. Its terminal elimination half-life may be prolonged to 22 hours. Clinical effects of overdose can include hypotension, tachycardia and drowsiness. A case report of overdose was published by Hustey[11] who recorded tachycardia, hypotension, prolonged QTc, and rapid progression to coma. Management involved activated charcoal, intravenous saline, and intubation for airway protection. The patient's mental status rapidly improved within several hours of the ingestion, and the prolonged QTc and tachycardia both resolved by the second and third days without further intervention.

Weight gain is a major problem with clozapine and olanzapine. Quetiapine has a favourable weight profile. In a study of 427 patients over one year quetiapine did not increase body weight, and had a tendency to shift the weights of underweight and overweight adults towards normal[4].

Quetiapine produces significantly fewer extrapyramidal side-effects than risperidone (odds ratio 0.39, $p = 0.0326$).

Bobes *et al.*[2] found that quetiapine was less prone to inducing sexual side-effects than either olanzapine or risperidone. In the so-called EIRE study, sexual side-effects were found in 35.3% of patients taking olanzapine and 43.2% of patients taking risperidone. Comparatively speaking, quetiapine only produced sexual side-effects in 18.2%. The conventional antipsychotic haloperidol produced sexual dysfunction in 38.1%.

Drug interactions

Phenytoin is a CYP3A4 inducer that may lead to an increase in the oral clearance of quetiapine if co-administered. Other hepatic inducers may produce similar interactions (for example, carbamazepine, phenytoin, rifampicin and barbiturates).

No interactions are seen with fluoxetine, lithium, imipramine, haloperidol, risperidone and lorazepam (single dose).

Conclusions

Quetiapine is an effective treatment for both positive and negative symptoms of schizophrenia, with similar overall efficacy to haloperidol and chlorpromazine:

- Quetiapine may improve mood in schizophrenia.
- Quetiapine has lower incidences of EPS than haloperidol, one of psychiatrists' favourite first-line treatments for schizophrenia.
- Quetiapine has a favourable weight profile.
- Quetiapine does not raise prolactin levels over those seen with placebo or produce frequent reproductive or sexual side-effects.
- No ECG, blood pressure or haematological monitoring required. Few drug interactions.
- Quetiapine has a very well-tolerated side-effect profile and, in long-term open-label extension studies, is associated with high levels of patient acceptability and satisfaction.

Quetiapine is an atypical antipsychotic that was launched in the UK in 1997. The clinical impression, post-marketing, is of a useful antipsychotic with few EPSs and with a potential to reduce positive and negative symptoms to a greater degree than some conventional antipsychotics. There is good tolerability in humans. Somnolence is the most common adverse event. Quetiapine appears to be less likely to induce sexual dysfunction than olanzapine, haloperidol or risperidone. Quetiapine has equal efficacy to risperidone in the treatment of schizophrenia, but produces fewer extrapyramidal side-effects. Quetiapine's general efficacy and side-effect profile suggest that, apart from any unforeseen post-marketing complications, it deserves a major place in the first-line and long-term management of schizophrenic disorders.

References

1. Arvanitis LA, Miller BG (1997). TI: multiple fixed doses of 'Seroquel' (quetiapine) in patients with acute exacerbation of schizophrenia: a comparison with haloperidol and placebo. The 'Seroquel' Trial 13 Study Group. *Biol. Psych.*,42(4):233–246.
2. Bobes J, Garc A-Portilla MP, Rejas J, Hernández G, Garcia-Garcia M, Rico-Villademoros F, Porras A (2003). Frequency of sexual dysfunction and other reproductive side-effects in patients with schizophrenia treated with risperidone, olanzapine, quetiapine, or haloperidol: the results of the EIRE study. *J. Sex Mar. Ther.*, 29(2):125–147, Mar–Apr.
3. Borison RL, Arvanitis LA, Miller BG (1996). ICI 204,636, an atypical antipsychotic: efficacy and safety in a multicenter, placebo-controlled trial in patients with schizophrenia. *J. Clin. Psychopharmacol.*,16(2):158–169.
4. Brecher M, Rak IW, Melvin K, Jones AM (2000). The long-term effect of quetiapine monotherapy on weight in patients with schizophrenia. *Int. J Psychiatry in Clinical Practice*, 287–291.
5. Copolov DL, Link CG, Kowalcyk B (2000). A multicentre, double-blind, randomized comparison of quetiapine (ICI 204,636, 'Seroquel') and haloperidol in Schizophrenia. *Psychological Medicine*,30(1):95–105,2000Jan.
6. Gefvert O, Bergstrom M, Langstrom B, Lundberg T, Lindstrom L, Yates, R (1998). Time course of central nervous dopamine-D2 and 5HT2 receptor blockade and plasma drug concentrations after discontinuation of quetiapine ('Seroquel') in patients with schizophrenia. *Psychopharmacol.(Berl.)*,135(2):119–126.
7. Goldstein JM (1998). Low incidence of reproductive/hormonal side effects with 'Seroquel' (quetiapine) is supported by its lack of elevation of plasma prolactin concentrations. Poster presentation,CINP.
8. Gunasekara NS, Spencer CM (1998). Quetiapine – a review of its use in schizophrenia. *CNS Drugs*,9(4):325–340.
9. Hellewell JSE, McKellar J, Raniwalla J (1998). 'Seroquel': efficacy in aggression, hostility and low mood of schizophrenia. Poster presentation,CINP.
10. Hirsch SR, Link CGG, Goldstein JM, Arvanitis

LA (1996). ICI 204,636: a new atypical antipsychotic drug. *Brit. J. Psych.*, 168(Suppl. 29):45–46.
11. Hustey FM (2000). Acute quetiapine poisoning [published erratum appears in *J Emerg Med* 2000 Apr; 18(3):403]. *Journal of Emergency Medicine*,17(6):995–7,1999Nov–Dec.
12. Kapur S, Zipursky R, Jones C, Shammi CS, Remington G, Seeman P (2000). A positron emission tomography study of quetiapine in schizophrenia: a preliminary finding of an antipsychotic effect with only transiently high dopamine D2 receptor occupancy. *Archives of GeneralPsychiatry*,57(6):553–9,2000Jun.
13. Kasper S (1997). Dopamine D2 receptor binding in typical and atypical neuroleptics. *Biol. Psych.*,41(75),67S(Abs227).
14. Langham S, McKellar J (1998). Patient satisfaction and acceptability of long-term treatment with 'Seroquel'.*ZenecaPharmaceuticals.*
15. Lieberman JA (1996). Atypical antipsychotic drugs as a first-line treatment of schizophrenia: a rationale and hypothesis. *J. Clin.Psych.*, 57 (Suppl.11):68–71.
16. Madhusoodanan S, Brenner R, Alcantra A (2000). Clinical experience with quetiapine in elderly patients with psychotic disorders. *Journal of Geriatric Psychiatry & Neurology*, 13(1):28–32,2000Spring.
17. Peuskens J, Link CG (1997). A comparison of quetiapine and chlorpromazine in the treatment of schizophrenia. *Acta Psychiatr Scand.*, 96(4):265–273.
18. Pollak PT, Zbuk K (2000). Quetiapine fumarate overdose: clinical and pharmacokinetic lessons from extreme conditions. *Clinical Pharmacology &Therapeutics*,68(1):92–7,2000Jul.
19. Purdon SE, Malla A, Labelle A, Lit W (2001). Neuropsychological change in patients with schizophrenia after treatment with quetiapine or haloperidol. *Journal of Psychiatry & Neuroscience*,26(2):137–49,2001Mar.
20. Reynolds GP, Tillery C, Elliott J, Blake TJ (1998). Human alpha2 adrenoceptor subtypes and their role in antypical antipsychotic drug action.Posterpresentation,CINP.
21. Small JG, Hirsch SR, Arvanitis LA, Miller BG, Link CG (1997). Quetiapine in patients with schizophrenia. A high- and low-dose double-blind comparison with placebo. *Arch. Gen. Psych.*,54(6):549–557.
22. Srisurapanont M, Disayavanish C, Taimkaew K (2000). Quetiapine for schizophrenia. *Cochrane Database of Systematic Reviews* [computer file]. (2):CD000967,2000.
23. Swerdlow NR, Zisook D, Taaid N (1994). 'Seroquel' (ICI 204,636) restores prepulse inhibition of acoustic startle in apomorphine-treated rats: similarities to clozapine. *Psychopharmacol. (Berl.)*,114(4):675–678.
24. Tandon R, Mullen J, Sweitzer D (2001). Quetiapine and risperidone in outpatients with schizophrenia: subanalysis of the QUEST trial. Poster presented at APA, New Orleans, 2001.
25. Vesely C, Kufferle B, Brucke T, Kasper S (2000). Remission of severe tardive dyskinesia in a schizophrenic patient treated with the atypical antipsychotic substance quetiapine. *International Clinical Psychopharmacology*, 15(1):57–60, 2000Jan.
26. Yeung P, Hellewell JSE, Raniwalla J, et al. (1998). 'Seroquel': extrapyramidal symptoms and tolerability profile in the elderly. Poster presentation,CINP.
27. Zarate CA Jr, Rothschild A, Fletcher KE, Madrid A, Zapatel J (2000). Clinical predictors of acute response with quetiapine in psychotic mood disorders. *Journal of Clinical Psychiatry.* 61(3): 185–9, 2000Mar.

Bibliography

1. Aizenberg D, Zemishlany Z, Dorfman-Etrog P, Weizman A (1995). Sexual dysfunction in male schizophrenic patients. *J. Clin. Psych.*, 56(4): 137–141.
2. Casey DE (1996). Side effect profiles of new antipsychotic agents. *J. Clin. Psych.*, 57(Suppl. 11):40–45;Discussion46–52.
3. Currier GW, Simpson GM (1998). Antipsychotic medications and fertility. *Psych. Serv.*, 49(2):175–176.
4. Ereshefsky L (1996). Pharmacokinetics and drug interactions: update for new antipsychotics. *J.Clin.Psych.*,57(Suppl.11):12–25.
5. Fabre LF, Arvanitis L, Pultz J, et al. (1995). ICI 204,636, novel, atypical antipsychotic: early indication of safety and efficacy in patients with chronic and subchronic schizophrenia. *Clin. Ther.*,17(3):366–378.
6. Fulton B, Goa KL (1995). ICI 204,636: an initial appraisal of its pharmacological properties and clinical potential in the treatment of schizophrenia.*CNSDrugs*,4(1):66–78.
7. Nutt DJ (1994). Putting the 'A' in atypical: does alpha-2 adrenoceptor antagonism account for the therapeutic advantage of new antipsychotics? *J.Psychopharmacol.*,8,193–195.
8. Schotte A, Janssen PF, Gommeren W, et al. (1996). Risperidone compared with new and reference antipsychotic drugs: *in vitro* and *in vivo* receptor binding. *Psychopharmacol. (Berl.)*, 124(1–2):57–73.
9. Wong JYW, Ewing BJ, Fabre LF, et al. (1996). Multiple-dose pharmacokinetics of 'Seroquel' (ICI 204,636) in schizophrenic men and women. *Eur.Psych.*,11(Suppl4),429S–430S.

Chapter 11
Focus on Amisulpride

Dr Ben Green

Summary

Amisulpride is a second generation antipsychotic, a substituted benzamide. Amisulpride appears to be an effective agent in treating schizophrenia for what are characterised as positive and negative symptoms. The recommended doses are between 400 mg/day and 800 mg/day. Amisulpride demonstrates a good global safety profile, particularly when compared with first generation antipsychotics, such as haloperidol. There are interesting studies that point towards amisulpride's antidepressant effect in dysthymia and one could speculate on possible roles in affective psychoses and chronic fatigue syndrome.

Introduction

Amisulpride is manufactured by Lorex-Synthelabo under the trade name Solian. Tablets are available in 50 mg or 200 mg formats. The recommended doses are between 400 mg/day and 800 mg/day. Amisulpride appears to be effective against negative symptoms at low doses – for example, 100 mg daily.

Indications

Primarily recommended by the manufacturer for the positive and negative symptoms of acute and chronic schizophrenia in adults.

As ever though, there are prescriptions of the drug outside licensed indications and there are reports of the drug's unofficial use for other conditions, even such apparently unrelated conditions as dysthymia[2,17].

Prescription for children and adolescents has been reported in the literature[18].

Pharmacology

Amisulpride has 'dual dopamine blockade' and a unique therapeutic profile being antipsychotic, at high doses, and disinhibitory, at low doses[16] – at low doses ($\leq$10 mg/kg) amisulpride preferentially blocks presynaptic dopamine autoreceptors that control dopamine synthesis and release in the rat; whereas at higher doses (40–80 mg/kg) postsynaptic dopamine D_2 receptor occupancy and antagonism is apparent. It binds selectively with a high affinity for human dopaminergic D_2 (K_i = 2.8 nM) and D_3 (K_i = 3.2 nM) receptors and is devoid of affinity for D_1, D_4 and D_5 receptor subtypes. It has no affinity for serotonergic alpha-adrenergic, H_1 histaminergic or cholinergic receptors. Amisulpride acts preferentially on presynaptic receptors increasing dopaminergic transmission at low doses[2].

There are two absorption peaks – one hour post-dose and a second 3–4 hours after taking the tablet. The elimination half-life is 12 hours.

Absolute bioavailability is 48%.

Amisulpride is weakly metabolised by the liver. There are two inactive metabolites. The drug is mainly eliminated unchanged by the kidney. 50% of an IV dose is eliminated by the kidney – of which 90% is eliminated in the first 24 hours.

Structure

Amisulpride is a substituted benzamide.

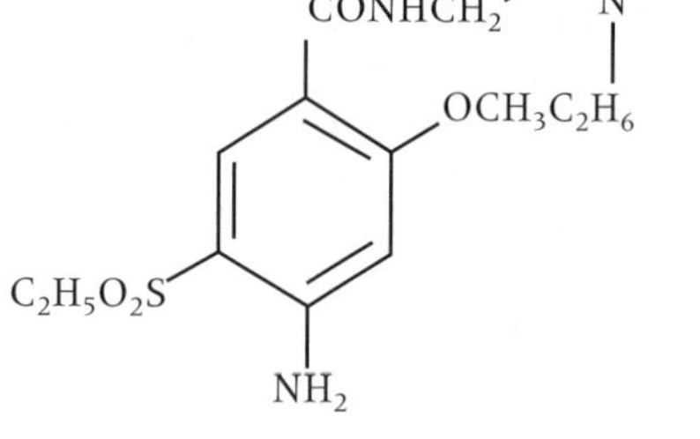

Figure 11.1: Chemical structure of amisulpride.

Efficacy

A four-week, double-blind, randomised study of 319 schizophrenia sufferers compared amisulpride with 16 mg haloperidol daily and found the efficacy was best at 400 mg to 800 mg daily (measured according to the Brief Psychiatric Rating Scale (BPRS) and the PANSS)[12].

Positive symptoms in schizophrenia

Wetzel et al.[19] compared amisulpride with flupenthixol – a conventional antipsychotic (a thioxanthene). The study ran for 6 weeks and involved 132 patients suffering from acute schizophrenia (DSM-III-R) with predominant positive symptomatology. Doses were initially fixed (amisulpride: 1000 mg/day; flupenthixol: 25 mg/day) but could be reduced by 40% in case of side-effects (mean daily doses – amisulpride: 956 mg; flupenthixol: 22.6 mg). Intention-to-treat evaluation demonstrated significant improvement under both medications. ANCOVA analysis showed that reductions of BPRS scores were more pronounced under amisulpride. Due to adverse events, significantly fewer amisulpride patients (6%) were withdrawn from the study (flupenthixol: 18%). Extrapyramidal tolerability was better in the amisulpride group.

Negative symptoms in schizophrenia

Amisulpride's efficacy against negative symptoms was investigated by Boyer et al.[1]. In this parallel group, double-blind, placebo-controlled trial, patients had to have high negative symptoms scores on the Scale for the Assessment of Negative Symptom (SANS) to be included. The authors said these were 'pure negative forms of schizophrenia'. 104 inpatients received amisulpride 100 mg daily, 300 mg daily or placebo. Amisulpride doses were significantly more effective on negative symptoms than placebo ($p < 0.02$). Interestingly enough, the differences between the 100 mg daily and 300 mg daily groups were 'minimal' according to the authors. Withdrawal symptoms from previous antipsychotics were controlled by a 6- or 12-week washout period.

Loo et al.[10] performed a multicentre, randomised parallel group, double-blind study looking again at fairly low doses (100 mg daily) compared with placebo. 141 patients received either amisulpride or placebo (69 receiving the drug). The study used SANS and Scale for the Assessment of Positive Symptoms (SAPS) on DSM-III criteria patients. All efficacy assessments were in favour of amisulpride.

Danion et al.[7] performed a placebo-controlled study of amisulpride on primary negative symptoms. After completion of a 4-week washout period, schizophrenic patients with primary negative symptoms participated in a 12-week, multicentre double-blind trial of placebo ($N=83$), amisulpride, 50 mg/day ($N=84$); or amisulpride, 100 mg/day ($N=75$). They were evaluated with the SANS, the SAPS, the BPRS, and the Montgomery–Asberg Depression Rating Scale (MADRS). Both amisulpride treatment groups showed significantly greater improvement in negative symptoms than the placebo group. The improvement in negative symptoms was independent of any improvement in positive symptoms.

Dysthymia

Smeraldi[17] reported a multicentre, double-blind, parallel group study in which 281 patients with DSM-III-R diagnosis of dysthymia or a single episode of major depression in partial remission were randomised and given either 3 months of treatment with amisulpride 50 mg/day or fluoxetine 20 mg/day. The baseline MADRS total score was reduced by at least 50% in 74.1% of patients (103/139) with amisulpride and 67.4% (87/129) with fluoxetine ($p = 0.230$). No significant differences between treatment groups were found in the reductions in mean total score with the MADRS, Widlöcher psychomotor retardation scale, Sheehan disability scale, and CGI. Anxiety measured by HAM-A total mean score decreased significantly more with amisulpride (63%) than with fluoxetine (54%; $p = 0.021$). There were 13 dropouts due to adverse events with amisulpride and 10 with fluoxetine. The number of patients reporting at least one adverse event was similar in the two groups (amisulpride 47.5%; fluoxetine 40.9%). As expected, in the amisulpride group endocrine-like adverse events in female patients were the most common, while nausea, dyspepsia, anorexia and insomnia occurred more frequently with fluoxetine.

Lecrubier et al.[9] compared amisulpride (50 mg /daily) to imipramine (100 mg/daily) in the treatment of patients with DSM-III-R criteria for primary dysthymia, dysthymia with major depression or major depression in partial remission. A total of 219 patients were included. Both analyses (intention-to-treat and 'per protocol' analysis) detected significant differences between groups (active treatment vs. placebo) on all main rating scales (CGI, MADRS, ERD, and SANS). The number of patients reporting at least one adverse event was higher in the imipramine group than in the two other, mainly due to anticholinergic effects.

Further work from this French group compared amisulpride and amineptine with placebo[2]. During this 3-month study of 323 patients, amisulpride (50 mg/day) was compared to amineptine (200 mg/day) in the treatment of primary dysthymia. Both amisulpride and amineptine were found to be statistically superior to placebo on the Clinical Global Impression (item 2), Montgomery–Asberg Depression Rating Scale and the Scale for the Assessment of Negative Symptoms.

This observed antidepressant activity was enthusiastically followed up by work such as that of Papp and Wieronska[11] who used two animal behavioural models: the forced swim test (FST) and the chronic mild stress (CMS) model. The duration of immobility time in FST was reduced by administration of imipramine (10 mg/kg) and amisulpride (1 and 3 mg/kg), although the effect of imipramine was more potent. In CMS, the stress-induced decrease in the consumption of 1% sucrose solution was gradually reversed by chronic treatment with imipramine (10 mg/kg) and amisulpride (5 and 10 mg/kg). The dosing appeared to be critical in that lower (1 or 3mg/kg) or higher (3 0mg/kg) doses of amisulpride were inactive. Amisulpride's onset of action was faster; at the most active dose of 10 mg/kg, amisulpride significantly increased the sucrose intake in stressed animals within 2 weeks of treatment while imipramine required 4 weeks before first effects on the stress-induced deficit in sucrose consumption could be observed.

These results provided further support for clinical observations that amisulpride may possess potent and rapid antidepressant activity.

Cautions and contra-indications

In the elderly amisulpride can cause hypotension and sedation. There are no systematic published data on efficacy in children less than 15.

Renal impairment significantly reduces the clearance and prolongs the elimination half-life of amisulpride and risperidone[4]. If there is renal insufficiency there should be a reduction in the dose of amisulpride. The dose should be halved if the creatinine clearance is between 30–60 ml/min. and reduced to a third for clearances between 10–30 ml/min.

Prescription should be avoided if there is proven hypersensitivity to the drug, a prolactin-dependent tumour, phaeochromocytoma, pregnancy or lactation.

Side-effects

Insomnia, anxiety, agitation are common side-effects (occurring in 5–10%). Somnolence, constipation, nausea, vomiting and dry mouth may occur in up to 2% of patients. Other side-effects include weight gain, acute dystonia, extrapyramidal side-effects, tardive dyskinesia, hypotension, bradycardia and QT prolongation.

Amisulpride can cause hyperprolactinaemia and thus may lead to galactorrhoea, gynaecomastia, breast pain and amenorroea. Amisulpride's endocrine effects are remarked on throughout the relevant literature. Gründer et al.[8] compared the endocrine actions of amisulpride and flupenthixol (a mixed D_1/D_2-like antagonist also blocking serotonin, H_1, and D_1 receptors) on anterior pituitary hormone secretion in schizophrenic patients. Blood was withdrawn at 15-minute intervals to assess basal secretion of prolactin, growth hormone (GH), and thyroid-stimulating hormone (TSH). Four hundred micrograms of thyrotropin-releasing hormone (TRH) was injected IV to investigate drug effects on TRH-stimulated secretion of prolactin, TSH, and GH. Prolactin plasma levels were markedly elevated in both treatment groups. This elevation was significantly more pronounced in females (but not males) with amisulpride than with flupenthixol. The prolactin response to TRH was significantly blunted by amisulpride only in male subjects. Interestingly enough, low basal prolactin levels predicted improvement of negative symptoms in patients treated with amisulpride.

Amisulpride may reduce reaction time in those using machinery. Seizure threshold reduction. May exacerbate Parkinson's disease. Neuroleptic malignant syndrome is a rare though possible side-effect.

The drug has been given to healthy volunteers and compared to haloperidol[14]. Amisulpride 400 mg daily had some mild adverse effects on psychomotor and cognitive performance, but no significant extrapyramidal disturbances in the group as a whole. On clinical rating scales or during a structured psychiatric interview it produced no signs of mental disturbances. Haloperidol ubiquitously impaired psychomotor and cognitive performance in a similar fashion after the first and the final doses and produced extrapyramidal disturbances in nearly every subject, the most common being akathisia and the most severe, in the case of one individual, being acute dystonia. Haloperidol produced a number of mental disturbances, the most noteworthy being negative symptoms.

Looking at the results from 11 studies Coulouvrat and Dondey-Nouvel[6] concluded that in these studies of a total of 1933 patients, amisulpride demonstrated a satisfactory global safety profile. There was an absence of cardiovascular events. Extrapyramidal side-effects were fewer than with haloperidol, endocrine events were similar to risperidone. Haematological and liver function problems were absent on laboratory tests. Their conclusion was that from a safety perspective amisulpride was superior to reference compounds.

Long-term safety data – Colonna et al.[5] – looked at 370 patients receiving amisulpride over 12 months compared to 118 patients on haloperidol. The overall incidence of endocrine events was comparable between groups (4% for amisulpride, 3% for haloperidol), but extrapyramidal events were predictably fewer in the amisulpride group. Maintenance of efficacy was comparable in both treatment groups.

Interactions

Co-administered ethanol increased the AUC by over 10%. There are no apparent interactions with benzodiazepines.

Since amisulpride is predominantly renally excreted, there is little potential for interaction with warfarin[15].

Comparison with other antipsychotics

Peuskens et al.[13] compared amisulpride with risperidone and found a marginal superiority for amisulpride. Their study was double-blind and involved 228 patients allocated, after a short washout period, to amisulpride 800 mg ($n=115$) or risperidone 8 mg ($n=113$) for 8 weeks. Decreases in mean BPRS total score were 17.7 ± 14.9 for amisulpride and 15.2 ± 13.9 for risperidone. All the individual factors on the BPRS showed a numerically greater improvement in the amisulpride group. There was a trend towards greater improvement in negative-symptoms patients receiving amisulpride. Patients receiving risperidone experienced an increase in body weight, which was significantly greater than for amisulpride ($p=0.026$).

Compared to the previous gold standard antipsychotic haloperidol, amisulpride has a superiority in treating schizophrenia in terms of positive and negative symptoms and a more acceptable side-effect profile[5]. Carriere et al.[3] found that compared to haloperidol, amisulpride had a beneficial effect on the quality of life measured by the Quality of Life Scale (QLS) and the Functional Status Questionnaire (FSQ).

Conclusions

Amisulpride appears to be an effective agent in treating schizophrenia for what are characterised as positive and negative symptoms (negative symptoms particularly at low doses – for example, 100 mg daily). Quality of life and function appears to be better on amisulpride than haloperidol. Furthermore, it appears to initially have a good global safety profile. There are interesting studies that point towards its antidepressant effect in dysthymia and one might speculate on possible roles in affective psychoses and chronic fatigue syndrome.

References

1. Boyer P, Lecrubier AJ, Peuch J, et al. (1995). Treatment of negative symptoms in schizophrenia with amisulpride. *British Journal of Psychiatry*, 166, 68–72.
2. Boyer P, Lecrubier Y, Stalla–Bourdillon A, Fleurot O (1999). Amisulpride versus amineptine

3. Carriere P, Bonhomme D, Lemperiere T (2000). Amisulpride has a superior benefit/risk profile to haloperidol in schizophrenia: results of a multicentre, double-blind study (the Amisulpride Study Group). *European Psychiatry: the Journal of the Association of European Psychiatrists*, 15(5):321–9, 2000 Aug.
4. Caccia S (2000). Biotransformation of post-clozapine antipsychotics: pharmacological implications. [Review] [191 refs] *Clinical Pharmacokinetics*, 38(5):393–414, 2000 May.
5. Colonna L, Saleem P, Dondey-Nouvel L, Rein W (2000). Long-term safety and efficacy of amisulpride in subchronic or chronic schizophrenia. Amisulpride Study Group. *International Clinical Psychopharmacology*, 15(1):13–22, 2000 Jan.
6. Coulouvrat C, Dondey-Nouvel L (1999). Safety of amisulpride (Solian): a review of 11 clinical studies. *International Clinical Psychopharmacology*, 14(4):209–18, 1999 Jul.
7. Danion JM, Rein W, Fleurot O (1999). Improvement of schizophrenic patients with primary negative symptoms treated with amisulpride. Amisulpride Study Group. *Am J Psychiatry*, 156(4):610–6.
8. Gründer G, Wetzel H, Schlösser R (1999). Neuroendocrine response to antipsychotics: effects of drug type and gender. *Biol Psychiatry*, 45(1):89–97.
9. Lecrubier Y, Boyer P, Turjanski S, Rein W (1997). Amisulpride versus imipramine and placebo in dysthymia and major depression. Amisulpride Study Group. *J Affect Disord*, 43(2):95–103.
10. Loo H, Poirier–Littre MF, Theron M, Rein W, Fleurot O (1997). Amisulpride versus placebo in the medium-term treatment of the negative symptoms of schizophrenia. *British Journal of Psychiatry*, 170: 18–22.
11. Papp M, Wieronska J (2000). Antidepressant-like activity of amisulpride in two animal models of depression. *Journal of Psychopharmacology*, 14(1):46–52, 2000 Mar.
12. Peuch A, Fleurot O, Rein W (1998). Amisulpride, an atypical antipsychotic in the treatment of acute episodes of schizophrenia: a dose-ranging study vs. haloperidol. The Amisulpride Study Group. *Acta Psychiatrica Scandinavica*, 98(1):65–72.
13. Peuskens J, Bech P, Moller HJ, Bale R, Fleurot O, Rein W (1999). Amisulpride vs. risperidone in the treatment of acute exacerbations of schizophrenia. Amisulpride study group. *Psychiatry Research*, 88(2):107–17, 1999 Nov. 8.
14. Ramaekers JG, Louwerens JW, Muntjewerff ND, *et al.* (1999). Psychomotor, Cognitive, extrapyramidal, and affective functions of healthy volunteers during treatment with an atypical (amisulpride) and a classic (haloperidol) antipsychotic. *J Clin Psychopharmacol*, 19(3):209–21.
15. Sayal KS, Duncan-McConnell DA, McConnell HW, Taylor DM (2000). Psychotropic interactions with warfarin. *Acta Psychiatrica Scandinavica*, 102(4):250–5, 2000 Oct.
16. Schoemaker H, Claustre Y, Fage D, *et al.* (1997). Neurochemical characteristics of amisulpride, an atypical dopamine D_2/D_3 receptor antagonist with both presynaptic and limbic selectivity. *J Pharmacol Exp Ther*, 280(1):83–97.
17. Smeraldi E (1998). Amisulpride versus fluoxetine in patients with dysthymia or major depression in partial remission: a double-blind, comparative study. *J Affect Disord*, 48(1):47–56.
18. Toren P, Laor N, Weizman A (1998). Use of atypical neuroleptics in child and adolescent psychiatry. *J Clin Psychiatry*, 59(12):644–56.
19. Wetzel H, Gründer G, Hillert A (1998). Amisulpride versus flupenthixol in schizophrenia with predominantly positive symptomatology – a double-blind controlled study comparing a selective D_2-like antagonist to a mixed D_1/D_2-like antagonist. The Amisulpride Study Group. *Psychopharmacology (Berl)*, 137(3):223–32, 1998 Jun.

Chapter 12
Focus on Ziprasidone

Dr Ben Green

Summary

Ziprasidone is a new antipsychotic with combined dopamine and serotonin receptor antagonist activity. The initial evidence suggests an effective dosage range of 80–160 mg/day. Clinical trials suggest that the drug is an effective antipsychotic in schizophrenia and schizoaffective disorder with a beneficial effect on negative symptoms and symptoms of depression. The main adverse effects appear to be somnolence (14%) and nausea (10%). Ziprasidone has relatively fewer side-effects and yet has at least equivalent efficacy for florid 'positive' symptoms compared to conventional antipsychotics. The additional serotonergic actions deliver further efficacy against 'negative' and affective symptoms of schizophrenia. Reduced effects on cognitive abilities compared to conventional antipsychotics make ziprasidone more attractive still. Barring any unforeseen complications it appears to a most valuable addition to the antipsychotic agents.

Introduction

Ziprasidone is a new antipsychotic with combined dopamine and serotonin receptor antagonist activity, developed by Pfizer[1]. Indeed its most potent action is action at the $5-HT_{2A}$ site. Ziprasidone has an *in vitro* $5-HT_{2A}$/dopamine D_2 receptor affinity ratio higher than most clinically available antipsychotic agents. Ziprasidone appears to have antipsychotic activity with a low liability for extrapyramidal side-effects[2]. Oral and intramuscular forms are available.

Dosage regime

Published trials have looked at the short-term efficacy of dosage regimes using 40, 80, 120, and 160 mg/day for schizophrenia and schizoaffective disorder[3,4]. Keck *et al.*'s trial looked at 139 patient randomised to receive ziprasidone 40 mg/day, 120 mg/day or placebo over 28 days[3]. It was the 120 mg/day dosage which proved significantly more effective against placebo. Daniel *et al.*'s study of over 200 patients demonstrated that both 80 mg/day and 160 mg/day were significantly better than placebo at reducing symptoms of schizophrenia with some antidepressant qualities as measured by the Montgomery Asberg Depression Rating Scale (MADRS) at 160 mg/day[4].

The initial evidence for an effective dosage range would appear to suggest prescriptions of 80–160 mg/day.

Oral and intramuscular forms of the drug exist. Rapid-acting intramuscular fixed doses of ziprasidone at 5, 10 and 20 mg have been well-tolerated[5]. These appear not be associated with extrapyramidal effects, dystonia or excessive sedation, but do control agitation[6]. The 10 mg dose appears to be clinically preferable[6a].

Structure

Ziprasidone* is a benzothiazolylpiperazine with the chemical formula:

$$C_{21}H_{21}CN_4OH . HCl)_2H_2O.$$

It is structurally dissimilar to its contemporary antipsychotics.

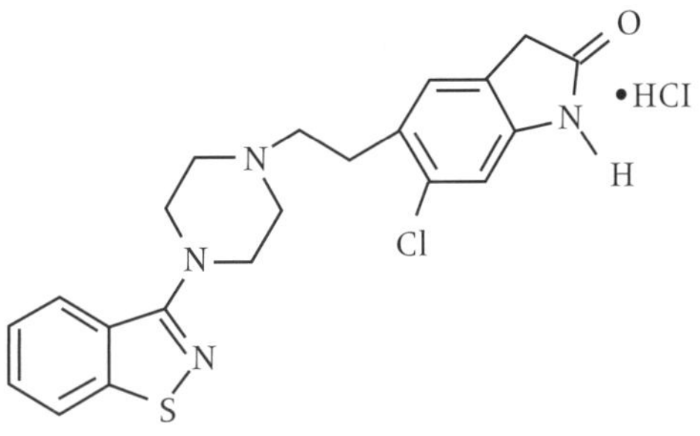

Figure 12.1: The ziprasidone molecule.

---

*5-(2-(4-(1,2-Benzisothiazol-3-yl) piperazinyl)ethyl)-6-chloro-1,3-dihydro-2(1*H*)-indole-2-one

Binding profile

Ziprasidone has pharmacologically important activity at serotonergic, dopaminergic and adrenergic receptors. This pharmacological activity led to early speculation that the agent might have antidepressant or anxiolytic qualities as well as antipsychotic potential[2]. Ziprasidone is a potent 5-HT_{2A} antagonist with an affinity for 5-H_{T2} receptors an order of magnitude greater than that observed for D_2 receptors. The emphatic antagonism of 5-HT_{2A} receptors in the brain may limit the EPS associated with dopamine receptor blockade and also improve efficacy against the negative symptoms of schizophrenia[1]. Ziprasidone also has high affinity for the 5-HT_{1A} (K_i = 3.4 nM), 5-HT_{1D} and 5-HT_{2C} receptor subtypes. Sprouse et al.[7] point out that ziprasidone's high affinity for 5-HT_{1A} is actually in terms of an agonist relationship, which differs from both clozapine and olanzapine and may produce clinical differences such as better anxiolysis or antidepressant action.

Ziprasidone is a less potent alpha-one antagonist than clozapine, risperidone, olanzapine and quetiapine It has less affinity for the H_1 and M_1 receptors than clozapine, olanzapine and quetiapine[8]. It may therefore have less potential for sedative side-effects than clozapine and olanzapine.

Initial researchers found that prolactin levels did not rise during initial treatment with ziprasidone for a month[9]. Later researchers have found transient rises though [10].

Ziprasidone's weak anticholinergic activity suggests a low potential for impairing cognitive abilities, which may indicate an advantage in the elderly who are prone to anticholinergic cognitive effects.

Clinical indications

In a double-blind study of some 200 or so patients on ziprasidone against 100 patients on placebo Daniel et al.[4] found that doses of 80 or 160 mg/day were statistically significantly more effective than placebo in improving the Positive And Negative Syndrome Scale (PANSS) total, Brief Psychiatric Rating Scale (BPRS) total, BPRS core items, Clinical Global Impression of Severity (CGI-S), and PANSS negative subscale scores ($p < .05$). Ziprasidone 160 mg/day was useful too for depressive symptoms and the authors inferred that ziprasidone was useful for acute exacerbations of schizophrenia or schizoaffective disorder.

The efficacy of ziprasidone against negative symptoms is further evidenced by a study by Meltzer et al.[11]. This randomised, double-blind, parallel group study of nearly 300 individuals was conducted at 26 centres. Measurements were made using the PANSS, Simpson-Angus and Barnes Akathisia scales, the Clinical Global Impression of Improvement (CGI-I) and the Abnormal Involuntary Movements Scale (AIMS). There was a significant ongoing clinical improvement in negative symptoms over one year, observable by 6 months of treatment.

Haloperidol has been the traditional treatment of choice for Tourette's syndrome, but this is an antipsychotic with a high potential for generating extrapyramidal side-effects (EPSEs). The early onset of Tourette's syndrome means that younger patients are therefore often exposed to antipsychotics such as haloperidol. An interesting pilot study by Sallee et al.[12] using ziprasidone for Tourette's against a placebo found that ziprasidone was well-tolerated and effective. It would be more interesting still to see a study that compared ziprasidone to haloperidol for this disorder.

Efficacy

Tuunainen et al.'s Cochrane review[12a] of the new antipsychotics (2000) erred very much on the side of caution and called for trials of sufficient power, with longer duration, measuring clinically important outcomes, to assess the true comparative clinical effectiveness, tolerability and cost effectiveness of newer drugs in relation to clozapine. Tuunainen et al. looked at 22 papers derived from 8 studies.

The specific Cochrane review for ziprasidone by Bagnall et al.[12b] cautiously concluded that ziprasidone may be an effective antipsychotic with less extrapyramidal effects than haloperidol, but it also may cause more nausea and vomiting.

Pharmacokinetics

Ziprasidone tends to show predictable linear pharmacokinetics. The mean C_{max} and AUC (0, 12 hours) increases with increasing dose, with apparent dose-proportionality between 20 and

Table 12.1: Main adverse effects with ziprasidone 80–160 mg/day in initial clinical trials[2].

Adverse event	Percentage of patients on ziprasidone (n=702)	Percentage of patients on placebo (n=273)
Somnolence	14%	7%
Nausea	10%	7%
Constipation	9%	8%
Dyspepsia	8%	7%
Akathisia	8%	7%
Dizziness	8%	6%
Diarrhoea	5%	4%

60 mg dose levels[10]. Steady state was achieved after one day. Trough-to-peak ratios at steady state ranged from 2 to 5. The dose of the drug does not need to be altered in mild to moderate renal impairment[13] or mild to moderate hepatic impairment[14].

Ziprasidone is highly protein-bound (>99%) and thoroughly metabolised with less than 1% being excreted unmodified in faeces or urine. There are no active metabolites.

There is little effect on cytochrome P-450 (CYP) isoforms. Ziprasidone is predominantly metabolized by CYP3A4 in human liver microsomes and is not expected to mediate drug interactions with simultaneously administered CYP substrates, at clinically effective doses[14b].

Adverse effects

Ziprasidone is generally well-tolerated[10]. The most frequent side-effects are mild or moderate headache. A minority of patients suffer first-dose postural hypotension because of alpha blockade. Ziprasidone is associated with a mild histaminergic sedative effect that becomes less pronounced as treatment continues. There are no drug-related changes in electrocardiogram or clinical laboratory variables reported. In Daniel's 1999 study[4] the percentage of patients experiencing adverse events was similar for 80 mg/day and 120 mg/day treatment groups, and resultant discontinuation was rare. The most frequent adverse events associated with ziprasidone in Daniel's study were generally mild dyspepsia, nausea, dizziness, and transient somnolence. Ziprasidone was shown to have a very low liability for inducing movement disorders and weight gain. According to Allison et al.'s meta-analysis study[18], weight gain attributable to ziprasidone therapy is only 0.44 kg on average. Taylor and McAskill's systematic review of 80 papers and reports concluded that ziprasidone did not appear to be linked to weight gain[9a].

Ziprasidone is associated with transient prolactin elevation, which is not dose-related, and which attenuates with chronic administration[10].

Some adverse effects traditionally associated with conventional antipsychotics, such as postural hypotension, were found to be very rare with ziprasidone.

Concerns about raised triglyceride levels with olanzapine and clozapine have led to interest in whether these characteristics are associated with other second generation agents. Ziprasidone in fact appears to be linked to a lowering of serum lipid levels[14a].

Interactions

There are no significant interactions with lithium although Apseloff et al.[15] did note a mean increase in serum lithium levels of 0.06 mmol/l in healthy subjects taking a moderate dose of lithium and ziprasidone. Induction of CYP3A4 with carbamazepine led to a modest reduction (<36%) in steady-state exposure to ziprasidone that is believed to be clinically insignificant[15a].

In terms of oral contraceptives, Muirhead et al.[16] found that ziprasidone could be administered with ethinyloestradiol and levonorgestrel without loss of contraceptive efficacy or risk of adverse events.

There is no interaction with aluminium and magnesium hydroxide antacids or cimetidine[2].

In a study on 24 extensive metaboliser subjects Wilner et al.[17] found that ziprasidone does not to inhibit the clearance of drugs metabolized by the 2D6 isoenzyme of cytochrome P450 (CYP2D6). Unlike clozapine and olanzapine ziprasidone is not metabolised by CYP1A2 and cigarette smoking (a CYP1A2 inducer) is unlikely to affect the metabolism of ziprasidone [2].

Comparison with other antipsychotics

Performance with regard to weight gain appears satisfactory compared to other antipsychotics. In a meta-analysis Allison *et al.*[18] found that whereas placebo was associated with a mean weight reduction of 0.74 kg, antipsychotics usually led to weight gain. Mean weight changes were as follows: thioridazine an increase of 3.19 kg, clozapine, 4.45 kg; olanzapine, 4.15 kg; risperidone, 2.10 kg; and ziprasidone, 0.04 kg. Their meta-analysis did not consider quetiapine.

The intramuscular form of ziprasidone is better tolerated in acute psychosis compared to haloperidol, which had a greater potential for acute movement disorders[19].

Cognitive functioning in a small, open-label, randomised trial indicated a trend towards better cognitive functioning in schizophrenia with one year's ziprasidone compared to risperidone. However, the small nature of the study really means that this is a potential area for more research, rather than an established finding[20].

Studies looking at switching from other antipsychotics have occasionally demonstrated improvements in psychopathology and negative symptoms, such as Daniel *et al.*'s study[21] looking at switching from olanzapine to ziprasidone in 58 outpatients over a short period. They found improvements in attention, vigilance, verbal learning and memory. Switching from conventional maintenance antipsychotics seemed to be associated with improvements in psychopathology, cognitive functioning and EPS (and consequent reduction in the need for anticholinergic medication) after 6 weeks of therapy with ziprasidone[22].

Conclusion

Ziprasidone is one of a new generation of antipsychotic drugs with relatively fewer side-effects and equal efficacy for florid 'positive' symptoms. The additional serotonergic actions of these new antipsychotics deliver further efficacy against 'negative' and affective symptoms of schizophrenia. Reduced effects on cognitive abilities compared to conventional antipsychotics make ziprasidone more attractive still. Barring any unforeseen complications, which become apparent after more widespread prescribing, ziprasidone appears to a most valuable addition to the antipsychotic agents. Health economic evaluations have yet to be published.

References

1. Seeger TF, Seymour PA, Schmidt AW, Zorn SH, Schulz DW, Lebel LA, McLean S, Guanowsky V, Howard HR, Lowe JA 3rd, *et al.* (1995). Ziprasidone (CP-88,059): a new antipsychotic with combined dopamine and serotonin receptor antagonist activity. *J Pharmacol Exp Ther*, 275(1): 101–13, 1995 Oct.
2. Tandon R, Harrigan E, Zorn AH (1997). Ziprasidone; a novel antipsychotic with unique pharmacology and therapeutic potential. *Journal of Serotonin Research*, 4, 159–177.
3. Keck P Jr, Buffenstein A, Ferguson J, Feighner J, Jaffe W, Harrigan EP, Morrissey MR (1998). Ziprasidone 40 and 120 mg/day in the acute exacerbation of schizophrenia and schizoaffective disorder: a 4-week placebo-controlled trial. *Psychopharmacologica*, 140(2):173–184.
4. Daniel DG, Zimbroff DL, Potkin SG, Reeves KR, Harrigan EP, Lakshminarayanan M (1999). Ziprasidone 80 mg/day and 160 mg/day in the acute exacerbation of schizophrenia and schizoaffective disorder: a 6-week placebo-controlled trial. Ziprasidone Study Group. *Neuropsychopharmacology*, 20(5):491–505.
5. Swift RH, Harrigan EP, van Kammen DP (1998). A comparison of fixed-dose, intramuscular (IM) ziprasidone with flexible dose, IM haloperidol. *European Psychiatry*, 13(4), S304.
6. Reeves KR, Swift RH, Harrigan EP, Lesem M (1998). Rapid acting, intramuscular ziprasidone 10 mg and 20 mg in patients with psychosis and acute agitation: results of two double-blind, randomized, fixed-does studies. Poster presentation.
6a. Lesem MD, Zajecka JM, Swift RH, Reeves KR, Harrigan EP (2001). Intramuscular ziprasidone, 2 mg versus 10 mg, in the short-term management of agitated psychotic patients. *Journal of Clinical Psychiatry*, 62(1):12–8, 2001 Jan.
7. Sprouse JS, Reynolds LS, Braselton JP, Rollema H, Zorn SH (1999). Comparison of the novel antipsychotic ziprasidone with clozapine and olanzapine: inhibition of dorsal raphe cell firing

and the role of 5-HT$_{1A}$ receptor activation. *Neuropsychopharmacology*, 21(5):622–31, 1999 Nov.
8. Pickar D (1995). Prospects for pharmacotherapy of schizophrenia. *The Lancet*, 345, 557–562.
9. O'Connor R, Harrigan EP, Heym J, et al. (1996). The efficacy and safety profile of a new antipsychotic, ziprasidone. Presented at the Xth World Congress of Psychiatry, 23–28 May, Madrid, Spain.
9a. Taylor DM, McAskill R, (2000). Atypical antipsychotics and weight gain – a systematic review. *Acta Psychiatrica Scandinavica*, 101(6):416–32.
10. Miceli JJ, Wilner KD, Hansen RA, Johnson AC, Apseloff G, Gerber N (2000) Single- and multiple-dose pharmacokinetics of ziprasidone under non-fasting conditions in healthy male volunteers. *Br J Clin Pharmacol*, 49(Suppl 1): 5S–13S.
11. Meltzer H, Arato M, O Connor (2000). Path analysis of the ZEUS study provides evidence of a direct effect of ziprasidone on primary negative symptoms in chronic, stable schizophrenia. *Schizophr Res*, 41 (1 Spec Iss):B91.
12. Sallee FR, Kurlan R, Goetz CG, Singer H, Scahill L, Law G, Dittman VM, Chappell PB (2000). Ziprasidone treatment of children and adolescents with Tourette's syndrome: a pilot study. *J Am Acad Child Adolesc Psychiatry*, 39(3):292–9, 2000 Mar.
12a. Tuunainen A, Wahlbeck K, Gilbody SM (2000). Newer atypical antipsychotic medication versus clozapine for schizophrenia. *Cochrane Database of Systematic Reviews* [computer file]. (2): CD000966, 2000.
12b. Bagnall A, Lewis RA, Leitner ML, Kleijnen J (2000). Ziprasidone for schizophrenia and severe mental illness. *Cochrane Database of Systematic Reviews* [computer file]. (2):CD001945, 2000.
13. Aweeka F, Jayesekara D, Horton M, Swan S, Lambrecht L, Wilner KD, Sherwood J, Anziano RJ, Smolarek TA, Turncliff RZ (2000). The pharmacokinetics of ziprasidone in subjects with normal and impaired renal function. *Br J Clin Pharmacol*, 49(Suppl 1):27S–33S.
14. Everson G, Lasseter KC, Anderson KE, Bauer LA, Carithens RL Jr, Wilner KD, Johnson A, Anziano RJ, Smolarek TA, Turncliff RZ (2000). The pharmacokinetics of ziprasidone in subjects with normal and impaired hepatic function. *Br J Clin Pharmacol*, 49(Suppl 1):21S–26S.
14a. Prakash C, Kamel A, Cui D, Whalen RD, Miceli JJ, Tweedie D (2000). Identification of the major human liver cytochrome P450 isoform(s) responsible for the formation of the primary metabolites of ziprasidone and prediction of possible drug interactions. *British Journal of Clinical Pharmacology*, 49(Suppl 1):35S–42S.
14b. Kingsbury SJ, Fayek M, Trufasiu D, Zada J, Simpson GM (2001). The apparent effects of ziprasidone on plasma lipids and glucose. *Journal of Clinical Psychiatry*, 62(5):347–9, 2001 May.
15. Apseloff G, Mullet D, Wilner KD, Anziano RJ, Tensfeldt TG, Pelletier SM, Gerber N (2000). The effects of ziprasidone on steady-state lithium levels and renal clearance of lithium. *Br J Clin Pharmacol*, 49(Suppl 1): 61S–64S.
15a. Miceli JJ, Anziano RJ, Robarge L, Hansen RA, Laurent A (2000). The effect of carbamazepine on the steady-state pharmacokinetics of ziprasidone in healthy volunteers. *British Journal of Clinical Pharmacology*, 49(Suppl 1):65S–70S.
16. Muirhead GJ, Harness J, Holt PR, Oliver S, Anziano RJ (2000). Ziprasidone and the pharmacokinetics of a combined oral contraceptive. *Br J Clin Pharmacol*, 49(Suppl 1):49S–56S.
17. Wilner KD, Demattos SB, Anziano RJ, Apseloff G, Gerber N (2000). Ziprasidone and the activity of cytochrome P450 2D6 in healthy extensive metabolizers. *Br J Clin Pharmacol*, 49(Suppl 1):43S–47S.
18. Allison DB, Mentore JL, Heo M, Chandler LP, Cappelleri JC, Infante MC, Weiden PJ (1999). Antipsychotic-induced weight gain: a comprehensive research synthesis. *Am J Psychiatry*, 156(11):1686–96.
19. Brook S, Krams M, Gunn KP and the Zirprasidone IM Study Group (1998). The efficacy and tolerability of intramuscular (IM) ziprasidone versus IM haloperidol in patients with acute, non-organic psychosis. *European Psychiatry*, 13(4):S303.
20. Hagger C, Mitchell D, Wise AL, Schulz SC (1997). Effects on oral ziprasidone and risperidone on cognitive functioning in pataients with schizophrenia or schizoaffective disorder: preliminary data. *Eur Neuropsychopharamacolgy*, 7(Isupl 2):219.
21. Daniel D, Stern R, Kramer T and the Switch Study Group (1999). Switching from olanzapine to ziprasidone: an interim analysis of a 6-week study. Presented at the 152nd APA. Washington, DC, 15–20 May 1999.
22. Weiden P, Simpson, G, Kramer T, Harvey P and the Switch Study Group (1999). Switching from conventional antipsychotics to ziprasidone: an interim analysis of a 6-week study. Presented at the 152nd APA. Washington, DC, 15–20 May 1999.

Chapter 13
Focus on Depot Antipsychotics

Dr Ben Green

Introduction

The use of depot antipsychotics is mainly a European phenomenon. The major reason for this is a belief in Europe that compliance is assured or improved with depots. Quite why they are not so popular elsewhere is difficult to say. Several depots are available in the UK. Haloperidol decanoate is available in the US.

In patients with poor insight and demonstrably poor previous compliance this may certainly confer benefit for the individual, the service and society. Depot antipsychotics have also been proven to reduce relapses, severity of relapse and reduce the frequency of hospitalisation[11,12,19]. Some individuals may also be prone to excessive first-pass metabolism and the depot's intramuscularly route of administration may bypass this problem. Overdose with antipsychotic drugs (except where iatrogenic) is obviously less of a problem too.

Care should be taken in switching from oral to depot formulations not to overdose the patient because of the absence of first-pass metabolism[22].

If adverse effects occur, however, they are naturally prolonged. This can prove problematic if dystonia or the neuroleptic malignant syndrome occurs.

Users sometimes perceive them as punishment for non-compliance or even other disagreements with staff. Particular side-effects include bleeding at the site, haematoma formation, and inflammatory nodules, which can be fairly common.

Administration can be enhanced by the use of a z-tracking injection[2].

Graphs of the plasma levels of the first dose of a typical depot show a similar profile with a sharp rise in the first 7 days with a peak thereafter and a gradual decline over the next 7–14 days. Chronic administration leads to more of a plateau, but there are still considerable variations with haloperidol decanoate and flupenthixol decanoate which may be associated with symptom breakthrough in some patients towards the end of a dosage period or if a dose is delayed.

To minimise side-effects and test for tolerability in the individual a test dose is often given and the patient's reaction observed over the next week.

The evidence-based literature for depot use is somewhat scanty, given their widespread use in the UK and Europe. Clinical decisions must largely be based on clinical observation, and are based on a literature often some twenty or so years old. Large-scale double-blind trials may not now be feasible without investment from state health systems, given that many of these older antipsychotic drugs are of limited profitability to the pharmaceutical companies. Such investment from health services might be warranted to establish a better evidence base.

Flupenthixol

Flupenthixol decanoate (also known as Depixol in UK) is a thioxanthene which should be administered every two to three weeks as a depot[6]. It is the most frequently prescribed depot in the UK. Peak levels occur 4–7 days after injection. It takes 10–12 weeks to achieve a steady state. A test dose of 20 mg may be given initially to assess tolerability.

Schizophrenia and schizoaffective disorders[16] appear to be the main indications for depot flupenthixol. Although psychotic conditions are the major use for this agent, there is recent interest in the use of oral flupenthixol for addictions (for example, alcohol[17] and cocaine[13]) and also for borderline personality disorder[15]. Oral use in affective disorders and in terminal care has also been documented[5,9,14] and also studied in anxiolysis[3] in where it was considered superior to beta blocker or placebo.

Depot flupenthixol has been trailed against oral amitriptyline and achieved similar efficacy, but the authors concluded that extrapyramidal side-effects would probably rule out its use except in tricyclic refractory patients[18]. The study involved only 68 outpatients.

A comparative study of depot flupenthixol with depot fluphenazine found that the former is less potent and that 25 mg fluphenazine decanoate corresponded to 40 mg flupenthixol decanoate[20].

Fluphenazine

Fluphenazine (also know as Modecate) is a potent phenothiazine administered every 1–3 weeks. It reaches its peak in 6–48 hours and takes 6–12 weeks to achieve a steady state.

A test dose of 12.5 mg may be used initially to assess tolerability. The dose can then be built up. Serum levels do not appear to correlate particularly with efficacy and so serum monitoring may not be useful in this regard[8].

In the same way that flupenthixol has been thought useful in borderline personality disorders, low dose fluphenazine has been found helpful in the management of multiple deliberate self-harm attenders, probably reducing self-harm behaviours[1].

Tardive dyskinesia may affect up to 50% of patients treated with fluphenazine.

Haloperidol

Haloperidol decanoate (also know as Haldol) is the decanoate ester of the butyrophenone haloperidol. It is one of the longer-acting depots and a month-long interval between injections is possible. It is available in sesame oil. Haldol reaches its peak in 4–9 days and takes 10–12 weeks to reach a steady state at monthly dosing.

Conversion from oral to parenteral form can be achieved by using an intramuscular dose 10–20 times the previous total daily oral dose. The initial dose should not exceed 100 mg.

In people who have not previously been on haloperidol a test dose might be given not exceeding 50 mg

Pipothiazine

Pipothiazine palmitate (also know as Piportil), a piperidine phenothiazine, is given monthly, reaches its peak in 4–10 days and takes 8–12 weeks to reach steady state.

Zuclopenthixol

Zuclopenthixol acetate (also known as Clopixol-Acuphase) is a short-lasting depot form of zuclopenthixol administered as 50–150 mg as a single dose. This provides rapid and effective reduction in psychotic symptoms in patients[24] over about 78 hours. It is often the drug of choice in acute psychiatric emergencies where organic factors are not paramount. A Canadian economic study showed a saving over haloperidol injection in some circumstances – for example, reduced nursing time and reduced repeat injections. Use in psychotic anxiety may also be possible[25].

Its duration of action is 2–3 days.

Although its main claim for use is in acute control of disturbed schizophrenia, the evidence base for its use over longer-established interventions is not particularly strong[7].

Zuclopenthixol decanoate (known as Clopixol or Clopixol Conc) is an established thioxanthene depot sometimes used in high doses where aggression is a problem, although it is not particularly licensed or indicated for this. It reaches its peak in 4–8 days and takes 10–12 weeks to reach a steady state at monthly dosing. It may be administered 2–4 weekly. Its efficacy appears to be similar to flupenthixol[4] and haloperidol decanoate[21].

As with other antipsychotics used, long-term monitoring of blood counts may be prudent as rare cases of neutropenia and thrombocytopenia may develop[10].

References

1. Battaglia J, Wolff TK, Wagner–Johnson DS, Rush AJ, Carmody TJ, Basco MR (1999). Structured diagnostic assessment and depot fluphenazine treatment of multiple suicide attempters in the emergency department. *International Clinical Psychopharmacology*, 14(6):361–72.
2. Belanger-Annable MC (1985). Long-acting neuroleptics: technique for intramuscular injection. *Canadian Nurse*, 81(8):41–3.
3. Bjerrum H, Allerup P, Thunedborg K, Jakobsen K, Bech P (1992). Treatment of generalized anxiety disorder: comparison of a new beta-blocking drug (CGP 361 A), low-dose neuroleptic (flupenthixol), and placebo. *Pharmacopsychiatry*, 25(5):229–32, 1992 Sep.
4. Dencker SJ, Lepp M, Malm U, (1980). Clopenthixol and flupenthixol depot preparations

in outpatient schizophrenics. I. A one year double-blind study of clopenthixol decanoate and flupenthixol palmitate. *Acta Psychiatrica Scandinavica, Supplementum*, 279:10–28.
5. Dwivedi VS, Berger AB, Khong TK, Hamilton BA, Jones PG, Brantingham P, Grillage MG, Prasad S, Kundu BN, Renwick JA, *et al*. (1990). Depression in general practice: a comparison of flupenthixol dihydrochloride and dothiepin hydrochloride. *Current Medical Research & Opinion*, 12(3):191–7.
6. Eberhard G, Hellbom E, (1986). Haloperidol decanoate and flupenthixol decanoate in schizophrenia. A long-term double-blind crossover comparison. *Acta Psychiatrica Scandinavica*, 74(3):255–62.
7. Fenton M, Coutinho ES, Campbell C (2000). Zuclopenthixol acetate in the treatment of acute schizophrenia and similar serious mental illnesses. [Review] [7 refs] *Cochrane Database of Systematic Reviews [computer file]*. (2):CD000525, 2000.
8. Gitlin MJ, Nuechterlein KH, Mintz J, Fogelson D, Bartzokis G, Ventura J, Subotnik K, Aravagiri M (2000). Fluphenazine levels during maintenance treatment of recent-onset schizophrenia: relation to side effects, psychosocial function and depression. *Psychopharmacology*, 148(4):350–4.
9. Gruber AJ, Cole JO (1991). Antidepressant effects of flupenthixol. *Pharmacotherapy*, 11(6): 450–9.
10. Hirshberg B, Gural A, Caraco Y (2000). Zuclopenthixol-associated neutropenia and thrombocytopenia. *Annals of Pharmacotherapy*, 34(6): 740–2.
11. Kane JM, Rifkin A, Quitkin F, Nayak D, Ramos-Lorenzi J (1982). Fluphenazine vs placebo in patients with remitted, acute first-episode schizophrenia. *Archives of General Psychiatry*, 39(1):70–3.
12. Johnson DA, Pasterski G, Ludlow JM, Street K, Taylor RD (1983). The discontinuance of maintenance neuroleptic therapy in chronic schizophrenic patients: drug and social consequences. *Acta Psychiatrica Scandinavica*, 67(5): 339–52.
13. Levin FR, Evans SM, Coomaraswammy S, Collins ED, Regent N, Kleber HD (1998). Flupenthixol treatment for cocaine abusers with schizophrenia: a pilot study . *American Journal of Drug & Alcohol Abuse*, 24(3):343–60, 1998 Aug. 98412970.
14. Lloyd-Williams M (1994). Treatment of depression with flupenthixol in terminally ill patients. *European Journal of Cancer Care (English Language Edition)*, 3(3):133–4, 1994 Sep. 95227445.
15. Kutcher S, Papatheodorou G, Reiter S, Gardner D (1995). The successful pharmacological treatment of adolescents and young adults with borderline personality disorder: a preliminary open trial of flupenthixol. *Journal of Psychiatry & Neuroscience*, 20(2):113–8.
16. Singh AN (1984). Therapeutic efficacy of flupenthixol decanoate in schizoaffective disorder: a clinical evaluation. *Journal of International Medical Research*, 12(1):17–22.
17. Soyka M, De Vry J (2000). Flupenthixol as a potential pharmacotreatment of alcohol and cocaine abuse/dependence. *European Neuropsychopharmacology*, 10(5):325–32.
18. Tam W, Young JP, John G, Lader MH (1982). A controlled comparison of flupenthixol decanoate injections and oral amitriptyline in depressed out-patients. *British Journal of Psychiatry*, 140:287–91.
19. Wistedt B (1981). A depot neuroleptic withdrawal study. A controlled study of the clinical effects of the withdrawal of depot fluphenazine decanoate and depot flupenthixol decanoate in chronic schizophrenic patients. *Acta Psychiatrica Scandinavica*, 64(1):65–84.
20. Wistedt B, Ranta J (1983). Comparative double-blind study of flupenthixol decanoate and fluphenazine decanoate in the treatment of patients relapsing in a schizophrenic symptomatology. *Acta Psychiatrica Scandinavica*, 67(6): 378–88.
21. Wistedt B, Koskinen T, Thelander S, Nerdrum T, Pedersen V, Molbjerg C (1991). Zuclopenthixol decanoate and haloperidol decanoate in chronic schizophrenia: a double-blind multicentre study. *Acta Psychiatrica Scandinavica*, 84(1):14–21.
22. Yadalam KG, Simpson GM (1988). Changing from oral to depot fluphenazine. *Journal of Clinical Psychiatry*, 49(9):346–8.
23. Yassa R, Iskandar H, Ally J (1988). The prevalence of tardive dyskinesia in fluphenazine-treated patients. *Journal of Clinical Psychopharmacology*, 8(4 Suppl):17S–20S.
24. Maragakis BP (1990). A double-blind comparison of oral amitriptyline and low-dose intramuscular flupenthixol decanoate in depressive illness. *Current Medical Research and Opinion*, 12(1):51–7.
25. Romain JL, Dermain P, Gresle P, Grignon S, Moisan P, Nore D, Pech G, Benyaya J, Perret I (1996). Efficacy of zuclopenthixol acetate on psychotic anxiety evaluated in an open study. *Encephale*, 22(4):280–6.

Chapter 14
Antipsychotics in the Elderly

Dr Emad Salib

Introduction

There is a range of widely differing drugs in this class. Each has an individual profile and, as a result, individual clinicians tend to get to know a few of the group and use these in preference to others. Antipsychotic drugs can be classified into:

1. Phenothiazines, aminoalkyl compounds (chlorpromazine), piperazines (trifluoperazine) and piperidines (Thioridazine).
2. Thioxanthenes (flupenthixol).
3. Butyrophenones (haloperidol and pimozide, a butyrophenone derivative).
4. Dibenzapines (clozapine).
5. Other newer agents: sulpiride (a substituted 0-anisomide), risperidone (a benzisoxazole), sertindole and olanzapine.

Pharmacokinetics

Actions:

- Block D_1 and D_2 dopamine receptors.
- Block 2 receptors.
- Anticholinergic.
- Antihistamine.
- Serotonin antagonism.
- Antiemetic.

Pharmacodynamics changes with aging result in a greater sensitivity of response to both the wanted and unwanted effects of neuroleptics[28].

In general, the phenothiazines are well absorbed, have substantial first-pass metabolism in the liver, and are widely distributed throughout the body. The have high tissue-binding and are slowly eliminated, and therefore have a relatively long duration of action. There is only mild enzyme induction. It is generally advisable to reduce the dose, at least initially, in elderly patients (especially in the physically ill) by about one-half to two-thirds of that used in the young. The various potencies and side-effect profiles of the phenothiazines make it possible for the clinician to make an informed choice to suit the circumstances. Age-related pharmacokinetic changes in drug disposition may result in higher plasma levels in elderly patients receiving the same dose as younger subjects (Jeste *et al.*, 1993)[15].

Side-effects of antipsychotics

To some extent, all antipsychotics block dopamine and produce varying degrees of extrapyramidal side-effects. The alpha-adrenergic blockage causes orthostatic hypotension and some sedation. Anticholinergic activity may lead to dry mouth, urinary hesitancy and possible overflow incontinence, constipation, and (to a lesser extent) blurred vision in the elderly. Paradoxically, the anticholinergic effects can be protective against extrapyramidal side-effects. A quinidine-like effect has been ascribed to phenothiazines, along with some direct myocardial depression which can, at high levels, precipitate cardiac failure. The cardiographic changes such as QT prolongation and inverted T and U waves are probably benign but in patients with myocardial disease and conduction defects, high dose should be avoided, especially with Thioridazine[4]. In the doses usually employed in the elderly, there are generally few toxic effects on the eye (for example, corneal or lenticular opacities) and retinal pigmentation is rarely seen. The skin in the elderly is seemingly more sensitive to the effects of neuroleptics, with an apparent increased incidence of slate-coloured pigmentation[8]; however, no evidence has been presented to show an increase in hypersensitivity or photosensitivity reactions. Clozapine can cause a serious granulocytopenia or agranulocytosis. Caution is necessary in patients with a history of myocardial disease (in particular with pimozide), hepatic disorder, prostastism and Parkinson's disease, but apart from agranulocytosis most contraindications are relative.

Table 14.1: *Side-effects of antipsychotic drugs (+++ marked, ++ moderate. + mild, + minimal, 0 none).*

	Antidopaminerfic	Antimiscarinic	Antihistaminic	Antialpha-adrenergic
Chlopromazine	++	+	++	+++
Thioridazine	+	++	++	++
Perhenazine	++	+	++	+
Trifluoperazine	+++	+	+	+
Haloperidol	+++	+	+	+
Pimozide	++	+	+	+
Sulpiride	+	+	0	0
Clozapine	+	+++	++	+
Promazine	+	+	+++	+
Risperidone	+++	0	++	+
Olanzapine	++	+++	++	+

Antidopaminerfic effects cause parkinsonism and akathisia. The former is a particular hazard in elderly patients. Lowering the dose, if practicable, is the first move; otherwise changing to a lower potency neuroleptic may help. Routine prescribing of anticholinergic agents to suppress such symptoms is not recommended as it may increase the risk of tardive dyskinesia in older patients[30]. Age is a major risk factor for tardive dyskinesia so that drug treatment should be reviewed regularly. Drug holidays can make the problem worse. Treatment of tardive dyskinesia is difficult, but sulpride benefits some patients[31]. Antihistaminic effects may lead to oversedation, especially when combined with other centrally active drugs, including antidepressants and hypnotics. Weight gain may occur with long-term use. Chlorpromazine is not a drug of first choice for the frail elderly. In addition, there are a number of idiosyncratic reactions of which the most important are the neuroleptics malignant syndrome, adverse side-effects (which are not confined to chlorpromazine) and agranulocytosis.

Extrapyramidal side-effects

Extrapyramidal side-effects do not seem to be related to antipsychotic activity. Thioridazine has fewer extrapyramidal side-effects, especially compared with the butyrophenones and those with an aliphatic side chain.

The 'atypical antipsychotics', such as Risperidone and clozapine, increase the ratio between antipsychotic activity and extrapyramidal side-effects, and may be of benefit in a minority of the elderly in whom parkinsonism or tardive dyskinesia is a significant problem.

Pseudo-Parkinson's disease

This is typically a triad of bradykinesia rigidity and (to a lesser extent) tremor. Although termed pseudo-Parkinson's the condition is quite similar to idiopathic Parkinson's disease. The likelihood of precipitating the condition rises with dose and remits with reduction of dose. They may be a delay in expression of the condition for up to years, but 70 per cent occur within 1 month and 90 per cent within three months of initiation[21]. The elderly, women, and those with organic brain disease are at greatest risk. Spontaneous improvement on stopping treatment is usually seen within a few weeks, although an unfortunate few remain symptomatic for years, and some exhibit signs again later in life. However, one must remember that there is a 1–2 per cent incidence of dyskinesia in the elderly.

The condition is helped by anticholinergic drugs such as Orphenadrine, Procyclidine etc. There is no advantage in using these drugs prophylactically, which cause additional anticholinergic side-effects and may increase the risk of later development of tardive dyskinesia[3]. Downward adjustment of the dose or a change to Thioridazine may be of benefit if the problem occurs. Anticholinergic treatment withdrawal may be attempted after 4–6 months. Amantadine can ameliorate the condition, but L-Dopa is not generally indicated for the treatment of pseudo-Parkinson's disease because dopaminergic drugs tend to exacerbate the psychiatric condition.

Tardive dyskinesia (TD)

Increasing age increases the likelihood of developing tardive dyskinesia whilst in psychotropic medication, and decreases the likelihood of recovery.

TD is a repetitive, involuntary movement of the tongue, lips, mouth, trunk and limbs secondary to drug use. If differs only in aetiology from idiopathic orofacial dyskinesia. Paradoxically, it not only appears whilst the patient is taking the neuroleptic but more commonly appears following withdrawal, even up to ten years later. It relates to the gradual loss of dopamine receptor blockade in the striatum, and the possible emergence of receptor supersensitivity. The prevalence increases with age, and it is more common in women. The repetitive chewing movements seen in otherwise normal elderly may be a subset of the condition. It is wise to exclude other coincidental causes such as the stereotyped movements seen in schizophrenia, focal dystonia, Huntington's disease, Wilson's disease, and rheumatic chorea. The duration of treatment is more strongly related than absolute dose to the emergence of the problem. Approximately 10–20 per cent of patients on a neuroleptic for a year or more develop appreciable symptoms. Plasma levels are not related. TD lasts for years, even after stopping the offending drug. Mehta *et al.*[22] showed that 11/13 elderly patients with TD had symptoms for over five years. Again, paradoxically, the treatment consists of cautious reduction (by approximately 10 per cent weekly) in stopping the offending drug, which unfortunately may worsen the psychiatric condition. Usually a month or two, but occasionally up to two years, may elapse before the symptoms abate. An attempt at control using another neuroleptic, such as pimozide, or by augmenting acetylcholine release with physostigmine can be tried. Clonazepam and lithium, along with many other medications, have been tried in this rather difficult condition. The best advice remains that prevention is better than cure, that is to say, restricting the use of antipsychotics to those clearly in need and using the minimum effective dose. Fortunately, the condition does not seem to be uniformly or relentlessly progressive, so the clinicians faced with a patient requiring a neuroleptic can be comforted by this fact; fortunately, the patient is rarely as concerned as the doctor or relatives. In summary, increasing age increases the likelihood of developing tardive dyskinesia whilst in psychotropic medication, and decreases the likelihood of recovery.

Akathisia

Because this causes restlessness with hand, finger, and foot movement it can be mistaken for agitation, but it is seen without autonomic disturbance or distress in the patient. The lack of response to anticholinergics, and the reduction in symptoms associated with a reduction of a neuroleptic, suggest postsynaptic receptor block-

Table 14.2:

Blockade of	Resulting side-effects
Dopamine	Extrapyramidal effects reports of dysphoria (unpleasant or low mood); agitation and anxiety.
Acetylcholine	Impaired cognitive function/confusion, dry mouth, blurred vision, constipation, retention of urine, fast heart rate.
Histamine	Sedation; also impaired cognitive function. Weight gain (but some evidence of weight loss in elderly).
Alpha-2 adrenaline	Falling blood pressure on standing (postural hypotension), hypothermia.
Other effects	
Effects on the heart	Impaired electrical conduction within the heart, with risk of abnormal heart beat.
Rare adverse events	Neuroleptic malignant syndrome (muscle rigidity, severe fluctuations of blood pressure and body temperature, with risk if death). Skin sensitivity and pigmentation (more common with high dose phenothiazines). Low white cell count (leading to decreased resistance in infections)

ade is the problem, possibly in the mesolimbic area.

Dyskinesia and dystonia

The classical oculogyric exaggerated posturing seen frequently in the young is rare in the elderly. It occurs soon after initiation of treatment and responds to anticholinergics.

Overview of antipsychotic side-effects

Interactions

Interactions which alter plasma antipsychotic levels may occur with: lithium, Phenobarbital, carbamazepine, phenyldantoin, cimetidine, propranolol and antidepressant drugs. Cost is a major issue with the newer agents such as risperidone and clozapine. Many clinicians have locally produced protocols for their use.

Clinical applications

Indications of antipsychotics in the elderly include: schizophrenia, paranoid disorders, affective disorders, disturbed behaviour, other conditions with mixed presentation and organic brain syndromes. The principles of treating schizophrenia and related disorders are similar at any age. Ageing results in reduced levels of dopamine and tyrolase hydroxlase, as well as lower counts of dopamine-rich neurons in the midbrain[5]. This raises susceptibility to neuroleptic-induced extrapyramidal symptoms.

Maintenance therapy

Post[25] suggested that only a third of patients with late paraphrenia, followed over 14 to 21 months, remained symptom-free. Regrettably, the advent of the newer antipsychotics and specialised services have not convincingly altered this prognosis[9]. Compliance, and therefore outcome, may be improved by the use of depot neuroleptics and the deployment of community psychiatric nurses.

All the current depot neuroleptics have been used in elderly patients and there is little to suggest that one is superior to another, or that any is less likely to precipitate parkinsonism. Dosages will generally be half that of younger adults. Parkinsonism may occur quite suddenly after weeks of treatment and may take months to wear off, or may expose latent Parkinson's disease. Many clinicians avoid the longer-acting depot agents (haloperidol decanoate, pipothiazine palmitate) in elderly patients.

In practical terms, the most important factor determining treatment response is compliance. Since patients are often socially isolated and typically insightless, adequate compliance with medication can often only be assured after hospital admission[27]. Post[26] predicted that the introduction of depot preparations of neuroleptics would make treatment failures rare by ensuring compliance. There is good evidence that, certainly in outpatient populations, use of a depot preparation rather than the oral route is associated with superior treatment response [9].

It is possible that an initial positive response to oral medication may encourage and motivate both the patient and clinician to proceed to a regular injection, and so prescription of depot medication may be an effect. The treatment

Table 14.3: Interactions with antipsychotics.

Drug group	Interaction with antipsychotics
Antidepressants	Metabolism may be inhibited, raising antidepressant levels.
Alcohol, barbiturates, other sedatives	Increased risk of over-sedation and slowed repiration.
Anticholinergic drugs (e.g. Procyclidine)	Reduced absorption due to slowed emptying of stomach; possible reduction of antipsychotic effect.
Antiparkinsonian agents	Reduction of antiparkinsonian effect.
Anticonvulsants	Increased enzyme activity (by anticonvulsants) may lower antipsychotic level.
Antihypertensives	Exaggeration of hypotensive (low blood pressure) effects
Antacids	Reduced absorption of antipsychotic

effects of an established relationship with a community worker should not be underestimated.

Depot injections

Although the use of long-term depot neuroleptic preparations overcome some compliance problems (assuming that patients make themselves accessible for injections and continue to consent to receive them), theoretically they may be associated with an increased risk of unwanted side-effects[2]. The evidence suggests that if low doses of depot medication are used and regular reviews for side-effects are carried out, then patients so treated may receive less total neuroleptic and experience fewer adverse events than if they had been treated with oral medication. In a study of the treatment of 20 chronic schizophrenic patients (mean age 63 years) with 12.5 mg of fluphenazine decanote every 21 days for six months Altamura et al.[2] presented an analysis of risk/benefit considerations. After 18 weeks of treatment, patients' total BPRS scores were reduced by 31.3% although there was no improvement in hallucinations. Some degree of rigidity was present in 90% akthasia and tremor in 50% and dysarthria in 35%. During the course of the study there were actually slight reductions in rigidity, tremor and dysarthria and the number of patients affected by akathisia fell by 20%. Extrapyramidal side-effects reached a maximal peak 36 hours after each of the first four injections, presumably reflecting early peak plasma concentration[1], but these were less prominent after the fifth dose, suggesting the development of tolerance. Reductions in measured supine and standing blood pressure were maximal in the first few days after each injection although this was not clinically significant.

The authors concluded that prescription of such low doses of depot medication had advantages over the oral medication regimens that these patents had received previously in terms of improvements in both efficacy and unwanted side-effects and a general reduction in the amount of neuroleptic administered. Howard and Levy[9] also reported use of lower total neuroleptic dose with depot rather than oral treatment. Late paraphrenic patients prescribed oral medication received on average a daily dose of 115 CpmqEq compared with 90 CpmqEq in those receiving a depot. Depot-treated patients also had lower total Abnormal Involuntary Movement Scale scores[32] than those receiving oral treatment.

Rapid tranquillisation

The elderly can become aggressive and agitated requiring emergency sedation. Clinicians should exercise more caution with sedation as coexisting physical illness may interact detrimentally with prescribed medication. For example, heavy sedation in a person with a confusional state secondary to cerebral hypoxia could be fatal. Bearing this in mind, the principles of rapid tranquillisation are the same as in younger patients, although doses need adjusting accordingly. Intravenous treatment is rarely required and intramuscular injections usually suffice. Prolonged and sustained aggression is not as often a management problem and hence long-term treatment is rarely necessary. Haloperidol is particularly effective at controlling aggression and a suggested regime for management is: (a) haloperidol 1 mg orally every hour (1–5 mg intramuscularly in an emergency); (b) continue with 0.5 mg to 2.0 mg, eight-hourly; when settled for 48 hours, reduce dose by 25%, continue with this until signs of aggression 'break through'; (d) aim to discontinue drug after a maximum of four weeks.

Agitated states and aggressive behaviour

Neuroleptics are moderately effective at reducing agitation and aggression. There is no established difference between Thioridazine and haloperidol. Lower doses are required than for treating psychoses in younger patients. In fact very low doses, such as 5 mg of Thioridazine, or 0.125 mg of haloperidol, may be effective. There is a concern that the anticholinergic effects of neuroleptics may contribute to cognitive decline in some patients with dementia.

The choice of neuroleptic depends upon individual preference and experience. Thioridazine is often prescribed but has marked anticholinergic effects. Haloperidol is another common choice but can cause extrapyramidal signs and symptoms. Sulpiride is useful when avoiding parkinsonism side-effects. Chloromazine is not recommended because of hypotension, and Promazine may be too weak. Regarding the newer agents, there are good theoretical reasons who clozapine may benefit patients with dementia with Lewy bodies. Risperidone and olanzapine may also be useful because of their side-effect profiles. Both clozapine and risperidone have been shown to be reasonably well tolerated and efficacious in psychosis in the elderly, and in the psychosis of Parkinson's disease[34,35]. The newer neuroleptics tend to be more expensive. Depot neuroleptics have been tried with some success and have the obvious advantage of improved compliance.

Use of the atypical antipsychotics

Because of its anticholinergic activity and relatively weak blockade of striatal dopamine D_2 receptors, low-dose clozapine may prove useful in the treatment of elderly psychotic patients who have individual sensitivity to extrapyramidal symptoms caused by typical neuroleptics[15]. Potentially confusing anticholinergic, together with hypotensice and sedating effects may, however, discourage widespread prescribing in this age group.

It is difficult to see how a drug which has been shown to impair memory function in young patients[7] will find favour with those who regularly prescribe for the elderly. Case-reports of individual elderly patients with functional psychoses which have been treated with clozapine are, however, generally positive.

Risperidone is a benzisoxazole derivative with extremely strong binding affinity for serontonin 5-HT_2 receptors, strong affinity for dopamine D_2 receptor and alpha$_1$ and alpha$_2$ adrenergic and histamine H_1 receptors[5,18]. Although clinical experience with risperidone in this patient group is extremely limited, activity at 5-HT_2 receptors appears to be important in the treatment of complex visual hallucinations[13] which are traditionally regarded as treatment-resistant[10,24].

Risperidone appears to be effective against hallucinations and delusions in elderly patients at very low doses (typically 0.5–2.0mg/day[13]). Hypersalivation is sometimes the only troublesome side-effect at such dosages although cases of the neuroleptic malignant syndrome have been reported[29].

Negative symptoms my occur in early-onset patients who have grown old. Since both clozapine[17] and risperidone[19,33] are effective in the treatment of negative symptoms, they may be indicated for the treatment of such patients.

In the absence of many reported studies involving elderly schizophrenic or delusional disorder patients, the treatment of drug-induced psychotic phenomena in Parkinson's disease (PD) with novel antipsychotics indicates that these drugs are tolerated by patients in this age group. Hallucinations and delusions appearing as side-effects of levodopa treatment in PD may be due to dopamine receptors[34]. Risperidone in very small doses (0.25–1.25 mg/day) improved hallucinosis in all of a group of six PD patients without worsening motor symptoms[35].

With the exception of clozapine and risperidone, which may have a part to play in the treatment of otherwise resistant symptoms, there is no real evidence that any particular drug is more effective in this group of patients.

Choice of drug for each individual patient should thus be based on considerations of concomitant physical illness and other treatments received, together with the specific side-effect profile of the antipsychotic[28]. Patients who do not respond to oral treatment (whether due to poor compliance or genuine treatment resistance) can be treated with a depot. Early-onset grown old patients do need bigger doses to control positive symptoms and there seems to be a wide variation between individual patients in the effective dose and tolerance of adverse side-effects.

There are some chronic graduate schizophrenics who need what are effectively young adult doses of neuroleptic to prevent relapse. This must certainly represent a group who are at particular risk of developing tardive dyskinesia[15] and who should be reviewed every few months by the prescribing psychiatrist rather than by a non-medical team member. In those patients who continue to experience psychotic symptoms after receiving depot for several weeks, the dose can be increased by 10% every two to three weeks until a response is seen or side-effects emerge. If this strategy is unsuccessful and if compliance with oral medication (and regular venepuncture in the case of clozapine) can be assured, then use of one of the atypical antipsychotics may be indicated.

Choice of a neuroleptic

As no ideal, or completely 'clean', neuroleptic is yet available, choice is a trade-off between antipsychotic advantage and likely side-effects. Since oversedation and, especially, EPS can cause particular problems in the elderly, anticholinergic (piperidine) side-effects are probably the best tolerated of the main three. Hence the popularity of Thioridazine.

Although pipothiazine (Piportil) is a depot Phenothiazine belonging to the piperidine group, there is no equivalent of decreased side-effects compared with either depot preparations to make this an inevitable first choice. In general the risk of serious side-effects with depot preparations in the elderly requires extreme caution do well on them. Careful monitoring is required. Parenteral phenothiazines, especially chlorpromazine, should be avoided in elderly people, because of the risk of potentially catastrophic hypotension. Intramuscular haloperidol is useful, both in calming aggression and in establishing treatment in those severely ill patients who are both non-complaint and without insight (and also perhaps liable to be detained under the Mental Health Act), the severity of whose symptoms requires urgent treatment. They can then be weaned on to oral medication, as both compliance and mental state improve. Such is the sensitivity of the elderly to even minor changes in dosage, great care is required to ensure that monitoring is adequate after discharge. Even in residential homes, unjustified assumptions are sometimes made about the competence of staff to judge whether a medication, perhaps written 'PRN', is really required, and in what dosage. This is a judgement taken more or less for granted by those with nursing or medical training, but many untrained staff, and carers, are simply not able to make it. Thus regular monitoring is required, by experienced workers who know the patient.

Even when successful control of symptoms, good compliance, and appropriate dosage have all been achieved, care is still required, especially in those living on their own, to avoid hypothermia, and the potentiation of other drugs such as analgesics and alcohol. Only one neuroleptic should be given at a time. Multiple prescription for the same patient is illogical, unnecessary, and tends to increase adverse rather than therapeutic effects. The aim should be to adjust the dose of one drug only, according to the patient's requirements and tolerance.

For similar reasons, prescription of antidepressants with maintenance neuroleptics in delusional disorders is to be avoided if at all possible. They may aggravate psychotic symptoms and increase anticholinergic side-effects and also be the wrong choice since apparently 'depressive' symptoms themselves need to be carefully interpreted: akinetic 'pseudodepres-

Table 14.4:

Drug	Potency eq. dose	Sedative effects	Extrapyramidal effects	Usual starting dose (mg)
Chlorpromazine	100 mg	high	moderate	10–25 bd/tds
Thioridazine	100 mg	moderate	low	10–25 bd/tds
Haloperidol	4 mg	low	high	2–3
Trifluperazine	5 mg	moderate	high	2–3
Thiothixine	5 mg	moderate	high	2–3
Pimozide	4 mg	moderate	high	1–2
Flupenthixol decanote		low	moderate	Approx. 20 mg
Fluphenazine decanote		low/mod	high	Approx. 12.5 mg
Clozapine	50–100 mg	high	very low	12.5 daily
Risperidone	2 mg	low	very low	0.5 bd

sion' required a reduction in the dose of neuroleptic or use if an anticholinergic drug, or both; difficulties in coping or factors such as loneliness, poverty, poor accommodation, or intolerance or rejection by family and friends required social intervention and practical help.

Anticholinergics should be used sparingly, and never routinely. Their toxicity in the elderly must never be under-rated. They may also precipitate tardive dyskinesia. They probably reduce both neuroleptic blood levels and clinical response. The emergence of EPS should, if possible, be treated by neuroleptic dose reduction initially, bearing in mind that the EPS may diminish spontaneously over a few months.

Key points in prescribing antipsychotics

Although the British National Formulary recommends that doses of neuroleptics in the elderly should be 25–50% of those given to young adults, elderly psychotic patients can often be effectively treated using neuroleptic doses which are much lower than this. Jeste et al.[15] have suggested that late-onset schizophrenics who have 'graduated' into old age are given higher doses of treatment than cases with onset in late life. Although late-onset patients may often be older than early-onset cases who have themselves grown old, such variation in age does not account for the differences in prescribed dose seen between these two patient populations. Jeste et al.[15] have suggested that late-onset schizophrenia is actually 'better prognosis schizophrenia'. In studies which have involved mixed late-onset and early-onset grown old schizophrenics, higher mean daily doses are reported than from the late onset or late paraphrenic studies. Jeste et al.[15] reviewed a group containing 25 late-onset schizophrenic and 39 early-onset grown old patients whose mean age was 59 years. These patients had been treated in an 'individualised', clinically optimal manner and received on average 443 CpmgEq per day. Prescribed medication dose was significantly higher in the early-onset group and correlated significantly with current age and age at onset. It would be useful to know which illness parameters are associated with poor response to medication. Pearlson et al.[23] found poor response to neuroleptics to be associated with (rare) presence of thought disorder and with schizoid premorbid personality traits. The presence of first-rank symptoms, family history of schizophrenia, and gender had no effect on treatment response. In a late paraphrenic patient group, Holden[12] found auditory hallucinations and affective features to predict a favourable response. This may, of course, simply reflect a better natural history in such patients.

With the exception of clozapine and risperidone which may have a part to play in the treatment of otherwise resistant symptoms, there is no real evidence that any particular drug is more effective in this group of patients. The choice of drug for each individual patient should thus be based on considerations of concomitant physical illness and other treatment received, together with the specific side-effects profile of the drug[28]. While there is an argument that all patients should be commenced on depot[27], treatment will usually be commenced at a low dose if an oral preparation (typically 0.5–1.0 mg of haloperidol or 10–25 mg of Thioridazine per day) which can be increased until a therapeutic effect is reached or side-effects develop. Patients who do not respond to oral treatment (whether due to poor compliance or genuine treatment resistance) can be treated with depot. Successful treatment of patients with depot can often be at very modest dosage. In those patients who continue to experience psychotic symptoms after receiving depot for several weeks, the dose can be increased by 10 per cent every 2–3 weeks until a response is seen or side-effects emerge.

There is no reason why patients in the community should not be maintained on depot for several years, so long as (and this is very important) they are monitored through examination by the prescriber for the presence of extrapyramidal side-effects at least once every 4 months in addition to regular reports from the nurse who gives the injection. If this strategy is unsuccessful, and if compliance with oral medication, then use of one of the atypical antipsychotics may be indicated.

Compliance with treatment is the most important determinant of outcome, while atypical neuroleptics are specifically indicated for patients with visual hallucinations or extrapyramidal symptoms. Elderly psychotic patients should be treated as vigorously and with as wide a range of neuroleptics as their younger counterparts and physicians should not restrict drug doses to modest levels in all cases so long as patients are monitored frequently for the emergence of side-effects.

Clinicians accept that treatment will lead to a remission or reduction in symptoms together with earlier discharge from hospital in most cases[28], but there is no agreement as to exactly how much improvement can be expected or in what proportion of patients it will be seen.

Because there are clear phenomenological, demographic and aetiological[36] differences between cases with late- and early-onset, and since early-onset patients who have grown old may have been receiving treatment for several decades prior to the period of study, these categories of patients are considered separately. Some authors have suggested a direct extrapolation of neuroleptic efficacy and response rated to the elderly from younger populations of early-onset schizophrenic patients[15].

One advantage of the methodologically weaker studies in late-onset patients, however, is that they have generally been able to report treatment success rates under essentially best clinical practice conditions. The most pessimistic and most optimistic estimations of the proportion of such patients who continue to experience psychotic symptoms, despite treatment, range from 73%[9] and 66%[25] to 52%[23] and 48%[37]. In early-onset schizophrenic patients, however, such inability to achieve complete symptomatic remission is less common, with figures of 25%[6] to 50%[16] typically quoted.

References

1. Altanura AC, Curry SH, Montogomery S, Wiles DH (1985). Early unwanted effects on fluphenazine esters related to plasma fluphenazine concentration in schizophrenia patients. *Psychopharmacoloft*, 87:30–33.
2. Altamura AC, Mauri MC, Girardi T, Panetta B (1990). Clinical and toxicological profile of fluphenazine decanote in elderly chronic schizophrenia. *Int J Clin Pharmacol Res*, 10:223–228.
3. APA (American Psychiatric Association) (1993) *Diagnostic and statistical manual of mental disorders*, 4th ed., APA, Washington.
4. Ballenger BR (1987). Antipsychotic agents. In *Clinical pharmacology in the elderly* (Swift CGH, ed.); pp. 434–64, Marcel Dekker, New York.
5. Cohen LJ (1994). Risperidone. *Pharmacotherapy*, 14:253–265.
6. Davis JM, Casper R (1977). Antipsychotic drugs: clinical pharmacology and therapeutic use. *Drugs*, 14:260–282.
7. Goldberg TE, Weinberger DR (1994). The effects of clozapine on neurocognition an overview. *J Clin Psychiatry*, 55(Suppl b):88–90.
8. Hader M (1965). The use of selected phenothiazines in elderly patients. *Mount Sinai Journal of Medicine*, 32:622–33.
9. Howard R, Levy R (1992). Which factors affect threatment response in late paraphrenia? *Int J Gerat Psychiatry*, 7:667–672.
10. Howard R, Levy R (1994). Charles Bonnet syndrome plus: complex visla hallucinations of Charles Bonnet type in late paraphrenia. *Int J Geriatr Psychiatry*, 9:399–404.
11. Howard R, Almeda O, Levy R (1994). Phenomenology demography and diagnosis in late paraphrenia. *Psychol Med*, 24:397–410.
12. Holden N (1987). Late paraphrenia or the paraphrenias: A descriptive study with a 10 year follow up. *British Journal of Psychiatry*, 150:635–9.
13. Howard R, Meehan O, Powell R, Mellers J (1994). Successful treastment of Charles Bonnet syndrome type visual hallucinosis with low-dose risperiodne. *Int J Geriatr Psychiatry*, 9:677–678.
14. Jeste DV, Harris MJ, Pearlson GD, et al. (1988). Late-onset schizophrenia: studying clinical validity. *Psychiatr Clin North Am*, 11:1–14.
15. Jeste DV, Lacro JP, Gilbert PL, Kline J, Kline N (1993). Treatment of late-life schizophrenia with neuroleptics. *Schizophr Bull*, 19:817–830.
16. Johnson EC, Owens DGC, Frith CD, Leary J (1991). Disabilities and circumstances of schziophrenia with neuroleptics. *Schizophr Bull*, 19: 817–830.
17. Kane J, Honigfeld G, Singer J, Meltzer H (1988). Cloprapine for the treatment resistant schziophrenic. A double-blind comparision with chlopromazine. *Arch Gen Psychiatry*, 45:789–796.
18. Livingstone MG (1994). Risperidone. *The Lancet*, 343:457–460.
19. Marder SR, Meibach RC (1994). Risperidone in the treatment of schizophrenia. *Am J Psychiatry*, 151:825–835.
20. Meco G, Alexandria A, Bonifati V, Giustini P (1994). Risperidone for hallucinations in levodopa-treated Parkinson's disease patients. *The Lancet*, 343:1370–1371.
21. Marsden CD, Tarsy D, Baldessarini RJ (1975). *Spontaneous and drug induced movement in disorders in Psychiatric aspects of neurological disease*

(Benson F, Blumer D, eds.); pp. 219–66. Grune and Stratton, New York.
22. Mehta D, Mehta S, Mathews P (1977). Tardive dyskinesia in psychogeriatric patients. *Journal of the American Geriatrics Society*, 25:545–7.
23. Pearlson G, Kreger L, Rabins P, *et al.* (1989). A chart review study of late-onset and early-onset schizophrenia. *Am J Psychiatry*, 146:1568–1574.
24. Post F (1965). *The Clinical Psychiatry of Late Life*. Pergamon, Oxford.
25. Post F (1966). *Persistent Persecutory State of the Elderly*. Pergamon, Oxford.
26. Post F (1980). Paranoid schizophrenia-like and schizophrenic states in the aged. In: Can schizophrenia begining after age 44? (Rabins PV, Pauker S, Thomas J (1984)). *Compr Psychiatry*, 25:290–293.
27. Raskind MA, Risse SC (1986). Antipsychotic drugs and the elderly. *J Clin Psychiatry*, 47 (Suppl 5):17–22.
28. Tran-Johnson TK, Harris MJ, Jeste DV (1994). Pharmacological treatment of schizophrenia and delusional disorder of late-life. In: *Principles and practice of geriatric psychiatry* (Copeland JRM, Abou-Saleh MT, Blazer DG. Eds.). pp. 685–92. Wiley, New York.
29. Webster P, Wijeratne C (1994). Risperidone-induced neuroleptic malignant syndrome. *The Lancet*, 344:370–1.
30. WHO (World Health Organisation) (1992). *The ICD-10 classification of mental and behavioural disorders*. WHO, Geneva.
31. Schwarts D, Wang M, Zeitel L, Goss ME (1962). Medication errors made by elderly chronically ill patients. *American Journal of Public Health*, 52:2018.
32. Schooler NR (1988). Evaluation of drug related movement disorders in the aged. *Psychopharmacol Bull* 24:603–607.
33. Hayberg OJ, Fensbo C, Remvig J, Lingjaerde O, Sloth–Neilsen M, Slavesen I (1993). Risperidone versus Perphenazine in the treatment of chronic schizophrenic patients with acute exacerbations. *Acta Psychiatr Scand*, 88:395–402.
34. Zoldan J, Friedberg G, Goldberg–Stenn H, Melaured E (1993). Ondansetram for hallicisis in advanced Parkinson's disease. *Lancet*, 341:562–563.
35. Meco G, Alessandria, Bonifati V, Giustini P (1994). Risperidone for hallucinations in levodopa-treated Parkinson's disease patients. *Lancet*, 343:1370–1371.
36. Castle DJ, Howard R (1992). What do we know about the aetiology of late onset schizophrenia? *Eur Psychiatry*, 7:99–108.
37. Robins PV, Pauken S, Thomas J (1984). Can schizophrenia begin after age 44? *Compr Psychiatry*, 25:290–293.

The author is most grateful for the support of Hollins Park Research Unit. To Janet Davies (Pfizer), Miss Katie Spencer and Ms. Susan Wright for their help in preparing the manuscript.